Cocaine in the Brain

MIND AND MEDICINE

Series Editors
Leonard S. Zegans, M.D.
Lydia Temoshok, Ph.D.

Previous volumes in this series

Emotions in Health and Illness
Theoretical and Research Foundations
edited by Lydia Temoshok, Ph.D.,
Craig Van Dyke, M.D.,
and Leonard S. Zegans, M.D.

Emotions in Health and Illness
Applications to Clinical Practice
edited by Craig Van Dyke, M.D.,
Lydia Temoshok, Ph.D.,
and Leonard S. Zegans, M.D.

Psychosocial Interventions with Sensorially Disabled Persons
edited by Bruce W. Heller, Ph.D.,
Louis M. Flohr, M.D.,
and Leonard S. Zegans, M.D.

Pychosocial Interventions with Physically Disabled Persons
edited by Bruce W. Heller, Ph.D.,
Louis M. Flohr, M.D.,
and Leonad S. Zegans, M.D.

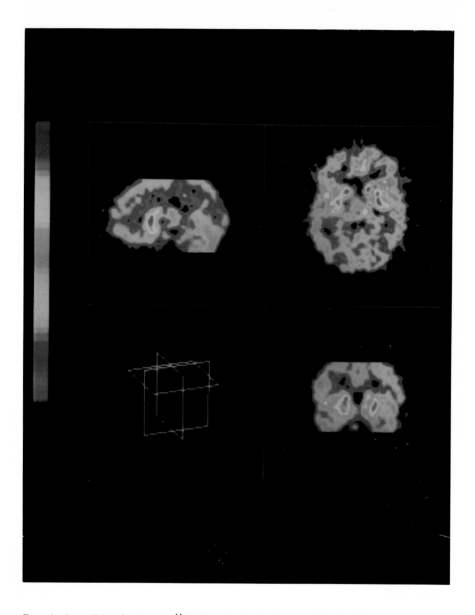

Frontispiece: Distribution of ^{11}C-Cocaine in the human brain. These images, obtained with a PET camera in a normal subject, represent three views of the brain: axial, sagittal, and coronal (clockwise from top left). The colors represent different concentrations of ^{11}C-Cocaine: the highest concentrations are shown by the red end of the spectrum, the lowest by the violet end (scale at left). Maximal concentrations of ^{11}C-Cocaine occurred in the caudate and putamen regions of the brain. Accumulations in these regions appear to reflect the binding of ^{11}C-Cocaine to the dopamine transporter (Fowler et al. *Synapse,* 4: 371–377, 1989). This work and material was done at Brookhaven National Laboratory with support from DOE-OHER.

Cocaine in the Brain

Edited by

Nora D. Volkow, M.D. and
Alan C. Swann, M.D.

RUTGERS UNIVERSITY PRESS
New Brunswick and London

Library of Congress Cataloging-in-Publication Data

Cocaine in the brain / edited by Nora D. Volkow and Alan C. Swann.
     p.   cm. — (Mind and medicine)
  Includes bibliographical references.
  ISBN 0-8135-1564-5
  1. Cocaine—Physiological effect. 2. Brain—Effect of chemicals
on. 3. Cocaine habit—Physiological aspects. 4. Cocaine—
pharmacology. I. Volkow, Nora D., 1956–   . II. Swann, Alan C.,
1946–   . III. Series.
  [DNLM: 1. Brain—drug effects. 2. Cocaine—adverse effects.
3. Substance Abuse.   WM 280 C65934]
  QP801.C68C627M1990
  616.86′4707—dc20
  DNLM/DLC
  for Library of Congress   89-70177
                                                 CIP

British Cataloging-in-Publication information available

Manufactured in the United States of America
The first three volumes in this series available from Grune & Stratton, Inc.
(Harcourt Brace Jovanovich, Publishers)

The editors and publishers gratefully acknowledge a publication subvention
from the Department of Energy–OHER.

Contents

Illustrations

Tables

Contributors

Edgar H. Adams, Sc.D.

Director, Division of Epidemiology and Prevention Research, National Institute on Drug Abuse, Rockville, Maryland

Burt Angrist, M.D.

Staff Psychiatrist, New York VA Medical Center; and Professor, Department of Psychiatry, School of Medicine, New York University, New York, New York

Charles Ashley, Ph.D.

Department of Psychiatry, State University of New York at Stony Brook, Stony Brook, New York

Charles A. Dackis, M.D.

Medical Director, Hampton Hospital, Rancocas, New Jersey; and Instructor in Psychiatry, College of Physicians and Surgeons, Columbia University, New York, New York

Everett H. Ellinwood, Jr., M.D.

Department of Psychiatry, Duke University Medical Center, Durham, North Carolina

Frank H. Gawin, M.D.

Associate Professor of Psychiatry, Substance Abuse Treatment Unit, School of Medicine, Yale University, New Haven, Connecticut

Joseph C. Gfroerer, Ph.D.

Chief, Statistical Analysis and Population Survey Section, Division of Epidemiology and Prevention Research, National Institute on Drug Abuse, Rockville, Maryland

Mark S. Gold, M.D.

Director of Research, Fair Oaks Hospital, Summit, New Jersey

Robert A. Hitzemann, Ph.D.

Department of Psychiatry, State University of New York at Stony Brook, Stony Brook, New York

Beatrice A. Rouse, Ph.D.

Chief, Epidemiologic Research Branch, Division of Epidemiology and Prevention Research, National Institute on Drug Abuse, Rockville, Maryland

Alan C. Swann, M.D.

Professor, Department of Psychiatry, University of Texas Medical School, Houston, Texas

Nora D. Volkow, M.D.

Associate Scientist, Medical Department, Brookhaven National Laboratory, Upton, New York

Roy A. Wise, Ph.D.

Center for Studies in Behavioral Neurobiology, Department of Psychology, Concordia University, Montreal, Canada

Leonard S. Zegans, M.D.

Professor and Director of Education, Department of Psychiatry, School of Medicine, University of California, San Francisco, San Franciso, California

Series Foreword

Several years ago, when the Mind and Medicine series was first conceived, the editors believed that there was a need for information about current research and its clinical applications concerning the connections between the psychological life of the individual and changes in body function. For many years there has been an artificial philosophical and scientific split imposed between the human psyche with its world of personal cultural meanings and the corporal realm of tissue and cellular activity. It has been difficult for the behavioral sciences to find ways of describing the essential unity of the human organism. Personal meaning was somehow not viewed as a salient biological phenomenon and the biochemical and molecular adaptations of the body were conceptually separate from the subjective life of the individual. Intellectually, we have been brought up in a Cartesian universe of dualism and we tend to think about issues of health and illness in a compartmentalized fashion.

Years ago, the "psychosomatic" movement tried to repair this split, but it was too heavily committed to a psychoanalytic model and found little place for the brain and its interactions with the rest of the body in its theory building. The editors of this series understand that it will be a long time before we possess an adequate model and language that could describe the complex interactions among environment, emotions and cognitive structures, the unconscious, neural networks, the neuroendocrine system, and the rest of the body. Yet in recent years exciting research has been progressing to construct experimental and conceptual links between these structures and processes within the body.

Past Mind and Medicine volumes have examined the role of the emotions in health and illness and then psychosocial approches to disabled persons. In planning our latest volume, we believed that there was no topic of more immediate concern to medicine, the behavioral sciences, and the public, than the issue of drug abuse, and, particularly, the misuse of cocaine. In exploring this topic we can begin to understand how the mechanisms of the neural receptor, the emotional world of the addict, and the social environment might be conceptually linked. We sought to produce a volume which both presented the most up-to-date research on brain mechanisms of cocaine use and examined this phenomenon from an historical/social and psychological perspective. Cocaine abuse cannot be understood from any one point of view. *Cocaine in the Brain* is intended to assist readers in comprehending the cocaine problem from multiple perspectives, which start from a base of knowledge about the neural mechanisms of craving and lead to new approaches to developing effective diagnostic, treatment, and prevention programs.

This volume defines our present knowledge about cocaine craving as a "biological phenomenon." But it also emphasizes how the memory of past drug-induced states and the "hope or expectation that this state might be produced again" help to explain the craving for this harmful substance. Thus we can understand how neuronal activity, memory, and the phenomenological state of the user sets the stage for a dangerous state of craving, which leads to the undesirable health and social consequences of cocaine abuse.

Leonard S. Zegans, M.D.

Introduction

Alan C. Swann and Nora D. Volkow

The effects of cocaine range from synaptic to cultural. The problems associated with cocaine use therefore combine neuroscience with social and political concerns. Cocaine acts on a system uniquely related to individual and social survival: neural reward. Teleologically, it would appear that the role of reward systems in the brain is to assure behavior necessary to the health of the individual and to the survival of the species. By acting directly on the system, cocaine first enhances other behaviors that produce reward, but can eventually supplant them.

This relatively simple formulation raises a number of questions: (1) Why have the social and epidemiologic problems associated with cocaine developed now and how is this related to the use of stimulants over previous millennia? (2) Why are these problems associated more with cocaine than with other pharmacologically similar drugs? (3) What are the effects of cocaine on the brain other than those on reward mechanisms, and what is their importance? (4) What are the long-term adaptations to repeated cocaine use, and how do they affect the systems on which the drug acts? (5) What treatment and preventive measures are most likely to be effective? This book will approach these questions using disciplines ranging from epidemiology to brain imaging.

Public concern about cocaine derives chiefly from the extent of personal and social disruption that results from its use or distribution: associated criminal activity, inability to work well, health problems, accidents, breakup of families. These problems can be examined using the methods of epidemiology and history. In the first chapter of this book, Burton Angrist examines the current problem of cocaine abuse in the context of previous "epidemics" of stimulant use. This approach provides useful information about the anticipated success of various measures to limit stimulant abuse, its consequences, and the overall natural course of periods of increased stimulant use. The second chapter, by Edgar Adams, Beatrice Rouse, and Joseph Gfroerer, examines the epidemiology of current cocaine abuse and the apparent trends in its incidence. This chapter also emphasizes the importance of combined abuse of cocaine and other drugs.

The study of the effects of cocaine on society must be accompanied by studies of its effects on the individual, (in particular, on the brain and behavior). In discussing the effects of cocaine in the brain, it is important to introduce two concepts that are crucial in understanding the reinforcing and addicting properties of cocaine. The first is its ability to block the reuptake of dopamine from the synapse; the second is the presence in the brain of several dopaminergic systems with different behavioral and adaptive properties. The ability of cocaine to inhibit neurotransmitter reuptake has been closely linked to its behavioral actions. Cocaine inhibits the reuptake of dopamine, norepinephrine, and serotonin with equal potency, but many of its behavioral and reinforcing effects appear to result from dopamine reuptake blockade. The diagram in Figure I.1 shows the role of reuptake blockade in transmitter function. The synaptic effects of dopamine, norepinephrine, and serotonin are largely terminated by reuptake of the transmitter into the nerve terminal. After reuptake, the transmitter is degraded into nonfunctional metabolites, such as the dopamine metabolites dihydroxyphenylacetic acid (DOPAC) and homovanillic acid (HVA). Reuptake blockade has two short-term effects: increased synaptic transmitter concentration and decreased production of certain transmitter metabolites. Over the longer term there are adaptations to these effects, as discussed in detail in Chapter 4.

There are several systems of dopamine neurons in the brain. Although these systems are similar in some biochemical and receptor characteristics, they differ in their behavioral and physiological effects and in the mechanisms by which they adapt to changes in activity. Figure I.2 is a schematic diagram of the major dopaminergic systems, showing the primary brain regions involved. As discussed in detail in the chapter by Roy Wise, cocaine's reinforcing properties largely involve the mesocortical system, which ironically

COCAINE AND DOPAMINE

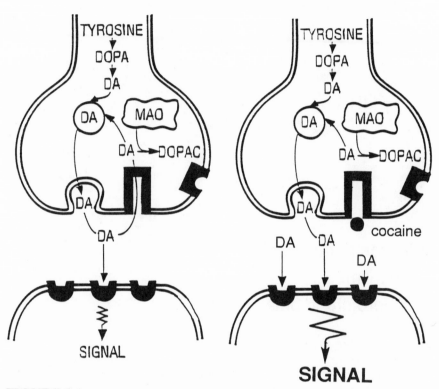

FIGURE I.1

Acute effect of cocaine on dopaminergic synapses.

The left half shows the drug-naive state, in which dopamine (DA) is synthesized from tyrosine via the intermediate l-dihydroxyphenylanine (l-DOPA). DA is stored in vesicles, released into the synapse, and elicits a signal by binding to pre-synaptic or postsynaptic receptors. The synaptic activity of DA is terminated by reuptake and breakdown via monoamine oxidase (MAO) and other enzymes to its metabolites dihydroxyphenylacetic acid (DOPAC) and homovanillic acid (HVA; not shown). The right half shows the effect of cocaine, which blocks the reuptake of DA, leaving more transmitter in the synapse for interaction with postsynaptic receptors.

Major Dopaminergic Pathways

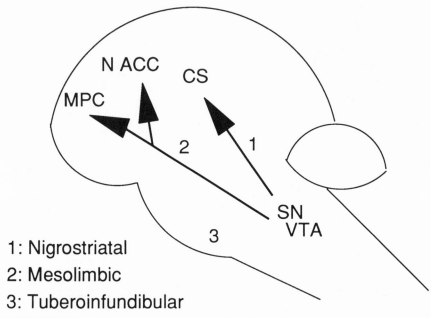

1: Nigrostriatal
2: Mesolimbic
3: Tuberoinfundibular

FIGURE I.2

Major dopaminergic pathways.
1: The nigrostriatal system consists of cell bodies in the substantia nigra (SN) and ventral tegmental area (VTA) of the midbrain with nerve endings releasing dopamine in the corpus striatum (CS). 2: The mesolimbic/mesocortical system consists of cell bodies in the SN and VTA with nerve endings releasing dopamine in limbic and cortical area such as the nucleus accumbens (N ACC) and medial prefrontal cortex (MPC). 3: The tuberoinfundibular system consists of cell bodies in the hypothalamus (arcuate and periventricular nuclei) with nerve endings releasing dopamine in the pituitary (neuro-intermediate lobe and median eminence).

has the least developed mechanisms for adaptations to changes in activity. This system has been implicated as having an important role in the mechanism of reward in the brain.

Cocaine's ability to stimulate neural reward mechanisms is evident from studies of animal and human behavior. If allowed to, animals will give themselves cocaine until they die. Animal experiments using intracranial self-stimulation, the ability to distinguish cocaine from other drugs, and self-administration of cocaine have produced important insights into cocaine's acute pharmacological effects. These methods can be combined with infusions of cocaine into selected brain regions, or with specific brain lesions or transmitter depletion; cocaine can be combined with drugs having specific antagonist actions in order to determine their specificity in terms of brain regions and transmitters. The possible biochemical mechanisms for these effects, and the resulting adaptations in the brain, are described in the chapter by Alan Swann. This chapter emphasizes studies of brain function, including measurements of transmitter synthesis, release, and uptake, receptor binding, and neurochemical events that follow receptor binding. Recent neurobiological evidence supports more complex effects than simple transmitter depletion. The complex interactions among the transmitters affected by cocaine are only beginning to be examined.

It is also becoming clear that cocaine affects different brain regions in markedly different ways. Such variations in brain function can be examined in vivo using imaging techniques. These include relatively static methods such as computer-assisted tomography and some applications of proton magnetic resonance imaging, as well as dynamic methods including measurement of cerebral blood flow, oxygen uptake, glucose metabolism, or receptor binding using positron emission tomography (PET). The chapter by Nora Volkow surveys the evidence that brain imaging offers about cocaine and brain function, concentrating on recent studies using PET on cerebral blood flow and glucose metabolism in chronic cocaine users. The data, although still preliminary, suggest that chronic cocaine use can impair brain function. An important locus of these effects is the medial prefrontal cortex, consistent with the behavioral and neurotransmitter effects described in the chapters by Wise and Swann. The recent development of selective PET probes for dopamine receptors and cocaine binding sites will provide the opportunity for a better understanding of the long- and short-term transmitter effects of cocaine.

The pharmacology of cocaine has an important influence on its effects in humans. The route of administration can affect the rate of onset and clinical characteristics of its effects. The rapid, intense reaction to "crack," a widely available form of cocaine that can be smoked, exemplifies the importance of examining the metabolisms and disposition of cocaine. This is the subject of Chapter 6, by shley and Robert Hitzemann. Information about the pharmacology of cocaine provides the basis for discussing clinical phenomena associated with its use.

The final two chapters of the book examine clinical aspects of cocaine use. The first, by Charles Dackis and Mark Gold, describes the pharmacology of cocaine including its neuroendocrine effects, medical complications, and pharmacological treatment. Finally, Frank Gawin and Everett Ellinwood, Jr., summarize the clinical phenomenology and natural history of cocaine abuse, its psychiatric complications, and their treatment. The newer pharmacological approaches are based on the behavioral and neuropharmacological data described earlier.

The chapters in this book take complementary approaches to several recurrent themes, including:

1. The disruptive power of reward stimulants (Chapters 1–3) and the tendency of society to oscillate between underreaction and overreaction (Chapters 1 and 2)

2. The role of dopaminergic systems (Chapters 3, 4, and 7), especially in the medial prefrontal cortex (Chapters 3–5), in acute reinforcing effects of cocaine

3. The complexity of transmitter interactions and adaptations to cocaine's effects, and the inadequacy of a single transmitter model despite its explanation of acute effects on reward (Chapters 3, 4, and 8)

4. The role of conditioning, and the riddle of apparent progressive sensitization to cocaine (Chapters 3, 4, 7, and 8)

5. The potentially severe medical complications of cocaine use (Chapters 5–8).

6. The development of treatments based on neurobiology (Chapters 7 and 8).

It is clear that new data in each field represented raise serious questions about views that have been taken for granted. Each field has an important contribution to the treatment of cocaine abuse and its associated problems. Chapters 7 and 8 describe encouraging short-term treatments for problems related to long-term cocaine use and withdrawal, based on the neuropharmacological effects described in Chapters 3 and 4 and pharmacology in Chapter 6. Successful long-term treatment, however, must depend on the ability of the individual to substitute experiential rewards for pharmacological ones.

1

Cocaine in the Context of Prior Central Nervous System Stimulant Epidemics

Burt Angrist

HISTORICAL PERSPECTIVE

Epidemics of central nervous system (CNS) stimulant abuse have occurred since the late nineteenth century. In this chapter these will be described only briefly, but references to more detailed historical accounts will be provided.

With the advantage of hindsight a rather characteristic pattern of events can be seen to follow the introduction of a new CNS stimulant: (1) Physicians explore the therapeutic potential of the agent, often enthusiastically. (2) Abuse occurs, the extent usually being in proportion to the drug's availability. This is often simultaneous with, not secondary to, the medical interest in the drug. (3) The drug is both publicized and viewed with some alarm. (4) Finally, when both the potential dangers and benefits of the agent are understood, specific medical indications for its use are defined. Abuse, if it becomes widespread, seems to decline only when the drug becomes less available.

This pattern of events was clearly apparent after the introduction of cocaine and elements of the pattern can be seen in the present cocaine epidemic. The same "story" was repeated, almost verbatim, after the introduction of amphetamine.

Cocaine, the First Epidemic

After cocaine was isolated in 1859–1860, discovery of its anesthetic properties enabled medical developments in ophthalmology and, shortly thereafter, in local and nerve block anesthesia. The central stimulant effects of cocaine appeared therapeutically promising, most notably to Freud, for treatment of depression and neurasthenia. The medical community recognized the potential of cocaine's stimulant effects to the secondary physical debility of other common medical ailments such as tuberculosis, and cocaine began to be used in a wide variety of such conditions. During this time cocaine appeared to be a "wonder drug." In July 1885, an editorial in *Lancet* noted: "The therapeutical uses of cocaine are so numerous that the value of this wonderful remedy seems only beginning to be appreciated." A possible literary consequence of this medical climate is that cocaine, prescribed for tuberculosis, might have led to Stevenson's creation of *The Strange Case of Dr. Jekyll and Mr. Hyde* (the interesting and extensive historical documentation of this possibility is presented by Schultz [1971]).

At this time, however, the drug was also freely available to the general population without a physician's prescription. Cocaine was advertised as a "cure" for virtually all problems and sold in a wide variety of unregulated (and unlabeled) home remedies and patent medicines. Coca tonics were endorsed by celebrities including intellectual, artistic, political, and religious leaders. Siegel (1985) has calculated that following the recommended regimens for such coca and cocaine products would have led to daily doses ranging from 20 to 1,600 mg.

The results of this free access were (now predictably) disastrous. Cases of addiction and psychosis were reported in the United States and Europe (Byck, 1974, 197; Jones, 1953, 94; Norris, 1901). In addition unpredictable reactions and deaths occurred after medical uses of cocaine both as a stimulant and as an anesthetic (Jones, 1953; Mattison, 1891; Woods & Downs, 1973) and cocaine rapidly fell into disrepute. Widespread abuse declined only after the passage of legislation such as the Pure Food and Drug Act of 1906 and the Harrison Narcotic act of 1914 in the United States and the limitations set on production and sale in Europe at the end of World War I. Some abuse of cocaine persisted, however, and prior reports of addiction, psychosis, and toxicity did not prevent the reemergence of widespread cocaine abuse in the 1970s. These "lessons" then had to be relearned.

More detailed discussions of the early history of cocaine can be found in Aldrich and Barker, 1976; Angrist and Sudilovsky, 1978; Byck, 1974; Jones, 1953; Peterson, 1977; Siegel, 1985; and Woods and Downs, 1973. Specific reports of addiction and psychoses from this period (in English) are: Gordon, 1908; Meyers, 1902 (cited in Siegel, 1985); Norris, 1901 and Owens, 1912. The most comprehensive historical references are Byck, 1974, and Jones, 1953.

The Amphetamine Epidemic

Amphetamine was first marketed in the United States in 1932 in the form of a nasal inhaler that contained 250 mg of racemic amphetamine (the Benzedrine inhaler). Abuse of such inhalers is a subplot in the general development of amphetamine abuse. The origins of this practice are unknown, but it was found that the containers could be broken open and the contents—an impregnated paper, or cotton pledget—extracted or swallowed. By 1947, in a now classic paper, Monroe and Drell found that 25% of prisoners in a military stockade abused amphetamine in this way. The Benzedrine inhaler was taken off the market in 1949 and the FDA banned amphetamine inhalers in 1959. A legal loophole left methamphetamine uncontrolled, however, and one company continued to market an inhaler (Valo) that contained 150 mg methamphetamine and continued to be abused, in some cases intravenously (Griffith et al., 1971). Abuse of inhalers containing mephentermine, which had psychotic sequellae, continued until 1970 (Angrist et al., 1972; Greenberg & Lustig, 1966), until these were removed from the market.

Amphetamine tablets were marketed in 1936 after Prinzmetal and Bloomberg (1935) demonstrated the efficacy of the drug in narcolepsy. Therapeutic applications of amphetamine were explored so enthusiastically by physicians that by 1939, Reifenstein and Davidoff reviewed "the current status" of "Benzedrine therapy" and cited 115 references describing applications in 22 conditions. By 1946 (Bett) amphetamine had been tried in 39 separate disorders.

As with cocaine, some patients tolerated high doses of amphetamine, whereas others developed severe reactions such as seizures and precipitous hypertension after modest doses (Reifenstein & Davidoff, 1939). The possibility of the drugs' being addictive was noted early by cautious investigators such as Guttman and Sargeant

(1937), Waud (1938), and Reifenstein and Davidoff (1939); but this was often strenuously debated. For example, Lesses and Myerson (1938) wrote, "As to addiction, the drugs to which human beings become addicted are the narcotics. There is no evidence in the entire literature of medicine that stimulants become habit forming." (Those who do not learn history are destined to repeat it.)

Abuse of amphetamine tablets was documented in 1937, in college psychology students in whom the effects of the drug were tested. Benzedrine (which was sold without prescription until 1939) was used in several colleges during the same year, as reported in *Time* magazine (1937). Amphetamine psychosis was first reported in 1938 (Young & Scoville) in narcoleptics; the authors noted that two of their three patients took larger doses than prescribed. "Benzedrine Benders" were described in the press and amphetamine tablets were called "brain," "confidence," and "superman" pills (Bett, 1946; Grinspoon & Hedblom, 1975; Snyder, 1974).

During World War II amphetamine was used by military forces on both sides. Grinspoon and Hedblom (1975) estimated that if 10% of American soldiers used amphetamine tablets "over 1.5 million men must have returned to this country with some firsthand knowledge of their effects." In the years following World War II media publicity continued and production of amphetamine increased to the point where it was measured in tons. In 1966 enough was manufactured to supply every man, woman, and child in the country with 35 doses (Sadusk, 1966). Amphetamine and related agents accounted for 6% of all prescriptions written (Griffith, 1966) and more than half the amount produced was diverted to the black market (Sadusk, 1966). In an exposé in 1964, for example, a CBS news producer set up a bogus "import-export" firm and used the letterhead to obtain more than a million doses of amphetamine and barbiturates from nine companies and suppliers (Grinspoon & Hedblom, 1975). Some polls reported that 20% of adults had taken amphetamine (Griffith, 1971), and polls of college students gave exposure rates that varied widely but averaged about 13% Berg, 1970; Gallup Organization, 1969). In the late 1960s high-dose, cyclic, intravenous amphetamine abuse and "speed" enclaves became established in San Francisco (Kramer et al., 1967; Smith, 1969) and New York (McNeil, 1967).

Parallel developments occurred in other Western countries. Connell's classic monograph from Great Britain, "Amphetamine Psychosis," appeared in 1958. One of its first conclusions was that "psychosis associated with amphetamine usage is much more frequent than would be expected from reports in literature." Kiloh and Brandon (1962) found that 3.4% of all prescriptions in one British city were for amphetamine preparations, representing approximately 2,600 patients taking an average of 77 tablets per month. Local physicians estimated that approximately 20% of those for whom the drug was prescribed showed some dependence. In the 1960s CNS stimulant epidemics were also reported in Scandinavia (particularly in Sweden [Inghe, 1969; Rylander, 1969]), Australia (Briscoe & Hinterberger, 1968), and Czechoslovakia (Vondracek et al., 1968).

The amphetamine epidemic in the United States ultimately ended for a variety of reasons. Legislation was passed that controlled the existing overproduction of amphetamine, physicians became more aware of the drug's dangers, and its legitimate prescription was limited to very specific conditions. (Further details on the epidemics of amphetamine abuse can be found in Angrist & Sudilovsky, 1978; Bett, 1946; Sadusk, 1966; Griffith, 1966; Griffith et al., 1971; Grinspoon & Hedblom, 1975; Monroe & Drell, 1947; Snyder, 1974.)

The Japanese Amphetamine Epidemic

A severe epidemic of intravenous amphetamine use occurred in Japan between the end of World War II and 1955. This was caused by "dumping" on the open market, soon after the war ended, stocks of amphetamines used by the military and by munitions workers. The amphetamine known as Zedrine and the more commonly used methamphetamine known as Philopon, Wake-amine, or Hospitan were freely available without prescription in ampule form and widely advertised to a demoralized population as providing "elimination of drowsiness and repletion of the spirit" (Hemmi, 1969; Masaki, 1956; Snyder, 1974). Each ampule contained 3 mg. The drug was usually taken intravenously in daily doses estimated as between 3–15 and 600–1,200 mg; the average daily dose was about 90 mg (Brill & Hirose, 1969). Use of the drug was originally noted in "the major commercial and industrial centers of Japan: Tokyo, Osaka, Kobe, Yokohama. From there, the drug spread to smaller towns and then to rural areas. Soon no prefecture in Japan was free of amphetamine addicts; Japanese law and practice defined addicts as persons who, of their own free will, are unable to give up the use of drugs" (Brill & Hirose, 1969).

By 1949 methamphetamine had been listed as a dangerous drug and its use was restricted by law. At approximately this time the first examples of "home brew" variety began to appear. These ampules varied in amphetamine content from none to 3.3 mg/ml. Bacteria were found in 45% of one series (Brill & Hirose, 1969).

The peak of the epidemic occurred in 1954, when Japanese users of Wake-amine numbered 500,000 to 1.5 million (from a total population of about 83 million [McConnell, 1963]), with half the users considered to be addicted (Masaki, 1956). More than 55,000 were arrested for violating the awakening-drug control law in that year; at least 10,000 were arrested in the months of May and June. In one slum area 10.2% of the bathers in public baths showed injection marks on their arms. A survey in the city of Kurume found that 5% of the population between the ages of 16 and 25 were Wake-amine addicts (Masaki, 1956).

In June 1954, the awakening-drug control law, drafted in 1951, was revised. The already severe penal clause was made even more so (Masaki, 1956), following which the epidemic dropped off sharply. By 1957 relatively few cases of amphetamine abuse were noted (Brill & Hirose, 1969; Hemmi, 1969).

THE CURRENT COCAINE EPIDEMIC IN THE UNITED STATES

The history of CNS stimulant abuse provides the context by which we can assess the current situation vis-à-vis cocaine in the United States. Most clinician–observers of drug abuse trends would agree with Wesson and Smith's (1985, p. 193) assessment:

Before the 1960's, when cocaine use was primarily associated with heroin and the hard-core drug culture, cocaine users were generally regarded as criminals. . . . But in the late 1960's and 1970's, many people changed their attitude about cocaine use. This attitude shift occurred for many reasons. Most important was a general

liberalization of attitudes about recreational drug use—a spinoff of wider accep-
tance of marijuana. Like marijuana, possession of cocaine was acknowledged to be
illegal but many people did not view its use as criminal. The media played a significant role. . . . Many people were taught to perceive cocaine as chic, exclusive,
daring and nonaddicting.

The lessons learned from the widespread cocaine abuse at the turn
of the century had been forgotten, and cocaine use began to increase
in the late 1960's and early 1970's.

Evaluation of trends of cocaine use since that time is invaluably
assisted by the availability of excellent demographic data that (to
this author's recollection) did not exist during the 1960s. Two such
studies, the National Survey on Drug Abuse (Abelson & Miller,
1985) and the Monitoring the Future Project (O'Malley et al.,
1985), closely replicated each other's data. Briefly, both studies documented precipitous increases in cocaine use, particularly by young
adults, between 1976 and 1979; from 1979 to 1982 all indices tested
(such as "ever" used, "used last year," or "used last month") remained stable, suggesting that during these four years enough new
users must have been recruited in the young adult age group to
replace those who moved out of it.

A quite different consideration is the consequences of this level
of use: What percentage of the 20–22 million Americans who report
"ever" having used cocaine will develop serious problems as a result? Clayton (1985), using what appears to be a conservative
method of estimating, has arrived at a figure of about 550,000.

Another approach is to apply data on longitudinal cocaine use
and progression of use to current demography. Such data are limited. In one valuable study Siegel (1985) followed 99 social-recreational users starting in 1974. In the first four years 8 stopped all
use, 41 dropped out, and the remaining 50 continued social-recreational use. Some of the last showed episodic patterns of more intensive use, but returned to their original use pattern. Over the next
five years, of the 50 subjects remaining in the study, half (25) continued social-recreational use (with episodes of increased use). The
other half showed some progression, with 32% (16) showing cir-
cumstantial (situation-linked) use patterns, 8% (4) becoming intensified (daily) users, and 10% (5) becoming compulsive uncontrolled
users. All of the last group had become freebase smokers. Thus for
the 99 patients initially enrolled, 8 stopped using cocaine and 41
dropped out during the first four years of the study, leaving their

status unknown; after nine years at least 25 had shown escalation of use pattern and at least 5 had become compulsive freebase smokers. If one applies these data to the National Survey on Drug Abuse figures for past month users only (4,160,000), one arrives at figures of 1,040,000 individuals who will shift into more intensive use patterns and 208,000 who will become compulsive users. These are probably very conservative estimates.

Still another approach to assessing the potential consequences of the current level of cocaine abuse is to consider the experience of cocaine treatment centers. Table 1.1 shows the rather homogeneous data from surveys done via the cocaine "hotline" in 1983 and 1984 (Gold et al., 1985) and from the Yale Cocaine Abuse Treatment Program (Gawin & Kleber, 1985). Table 1.2 is included only to emphasize the severity of the problems reported by individuals requesting treatment for cocaine dependence via the cocaine hotline (Gold et al., 1985).

A point to emphasize in Table 1.1 is that these individuals found it necessary to seek treatment after *mean* durations of cocaine use ranging from 3.5 to 4.8 years (with large variance). In this context a point made by Clayton (1983, 1985, p. 30) deserves emphasis: "It may well be true that the increases in the number of clients seeking treatment for cocaine represents the *front* end of a longer line of people. These are the people who have used cocaine long enough to

TABLE 1.1

Characteristics of Cocaine Abusers Requesting Treatment

	Yale cocaine abuse treatment program	Cocaine "hotline"	
		1983	1984
Age	28.6	31	28.5
Route			
Intranasal	37%	58%	60%
Intravenous	43%	26%	13%
Smoking	20%	16%	27%
Dose (gm/week)	6.1	5.5	6.2
Duration of use (yrs)	4.8	4.6	3.5

SOURCE: Gawin and Kleber (1985) and Gold et al. (1985).

TABLE 1.2
Adverse Social and Other Effects Reported by 200 Callers to Cocaine
"Hotline" in 1983 and 1984

	1983	1984
Dealing cocaine to support habit	43%	47%
Stealing from work	20%	28%
Stealing from family or friends	28%	42%
Arrested for dealing or possession	17%	14%
Automobile accident on cocaine	9%	39%
Loss of job due to cocaine	16%	15%
Loss of spouse due to cocaine	30%	33%
In debt due to cocaine	46%	57%

SOURCE: Gold et al. (1985).

progress far enough to have problems. If the average hiatus is from 3–5 years, the appearance of large numbers of new cases in treatment centers may be imminent."

Another major cause for concern is the frequency with which intensive routes of administration such as freebase smoking and intravenous use are being reported. The precipitous rise of psychostimulant plasma levels associated with such routes of administration causes effects that are profoundly reinforcing. An example is Rylander's (1969, p. 254) description of the effects of high-dose intravenous phenmetrazine: "One of the addicts . . . said that at first he feels numb and, if he is standing, he goes down on his knees. The heart starts beating at a terrible speed and his respiration is very rapid. Then he feels as if he were ascending into the cosmos, every fiber of his body trembling with happiness."

This experience, called the "rush," and often explicitly compared to a total body orgasm, is a highly prized and psychologically potent effect that may profoundly alter much of a user's subsequent pattern of drug use. This occurs, first, because the effect becomes autonomously desired (i.e., over and above the stimulant effects that persist after the "rush" abates), predisposing the user to repeated injections (or, with cocaine base, smoking) and a cyclic "binge" pattern of use. Second, repeated doses may be taken at a time when an oral or intranasal user might judge that he or she has "had enough," leading to increased cumulative doses and greater risk of psychosis, physical toxicity, and severe depressive "crash-ing" syndromes. Finally, these profoundly reinforcing effects in-duce a proportionately severe degree of dependence. Virtually all clinical investigators of CNS stimulants concur on this point. Ka-lant (1973) explicitly noted that "the rate and strength of develop-ment of psychological dependence was intensified by intravenous use." Both Siegel (1979) and Van Dyke and Byck (1982) have stressed the importance of smoking and injection as a determinant of severe cocaine dependence. In the longitudinal study of initially recreational users cited earlier (Siegel, 1985) all of those who be-came compulsive users had been smoking cocaine base.

A particularly dramatic demonstration of the dangers of cocaine freebase smoking occurred after the introduction of "crack" in the Bahamas. Jekel et al. (1986, pp. 461, 459) reported that former ad-dicts confirmed:

that cocaine powder had been available, if expensive, for years, but that in late 1982 or early 1983 the drug suddenly became much more plentiful as production in South America increased. The street price of cocaine in Nassau fell to one–fifth of its former level.

Ex–addicts also told us that at about the time that cocaine became more plenti-ful and cheaper drug pushers switched from selling powdered cocaine ("snow") for nasal inhalation or injection to the pure alkaloid form ("rocks" or "freebase") which is used exclusively for smoking. It suddenly became very difficult to obtain powder in Nassau. By making this change, the drug pushers were forcing all co-caine users to become addicts. . . . Selling freebase guarantees an eager market for the increasingly available cocaine.

In the context of these developments cocaine–related psychiatric admissions increased from "none in 1982 to 69 in 1983 and to 523 in 1984." The clinical spectrum was described (Jekel et al., 1986, p. 461) as follows:

The cocaine addicts often presented with severe depression, manifest by unkempt appearance, insomnia, anorexia, withdrawal, and suicidal ideation. There were at least 10 cocaine-associated deaths, 5 of which were suicides. Cocaine psychosis was common: the patient would present with severe agitation, impired judgement, paranoid ideation, intense denial, violent behaviour, threats of suicide or homicide, and hallucinations. In periods of lucidity they would try to mislead the physician, and a relative or friend was needed to confirm the psychotic state.

Physical problems associated with the intensity of abuse were als prominent and included seizures, cardiac arrhythmia, pneumonia, avitaminosis, and severe malnutrition. A similar spectrum of clinical effects, that is, severe dependence and psychiatric sequelae and potentially serious medical problems, has been seen in the cocaine-producing countries of South America after the smoking of cocaine paste (Erickson et al., 1987; Jeri, 1984).

Another lesson from the past (that offers little comfort) is that stimulant epidemics were in large part controlled by reducing supplies. For example, in the United States amphetamine overproduction by drug companies could directly be controlled by legislation. In the case of the multimillion dollar, criminal, cocaine "industry," however, control is easier to propose than to achieve. Decreasing costs and increasing purity of seized samples are also of concern (Clayton, 1985).

In summary, then, cocaine is likely to remain a significant problem in the United States. Its use is widely established in the population, creating a large market, and suppliers of that market are unlikely to be combated with complete success. Highly reinforcing routes of administration are reported frequently and these users are at high risk for developing severe dependence. The trends seen in treatment programs cannot be reversed quickly.

The only optimistic aspects of the current situation are (1) the progress being made in development of potential pharmacological treatments for cocaine dependence (Gawin, 1986) and (2) the efforts to increase general awareness of the negative consequences of cocaine use. Only future epidemiological data will determine the impact of the latter factor.

DIFFERENTIAL INCIDENCE OF PSYCHOSIS AFTER COCAINE AND AMPHETAMINE?

When amphetamine was widely abused, amphetamine psychosis was a frequent occurrence. For example, in her review of the medical literature from 1938 to 1963, Kalant (1973) documented more than 60 reports of psychoses following acute or chronic amphetamine use. Moreover, in studies in which amphetamine psychosis was prospectively induced experimentally in nonpsychotic abusers, 25 of 32 subjects ultimately developed a psychosis (Angrist & Gershon, 1970; Angrist et al., 1972; Bell, 1973; Griffith et al., 1968, 1972).

In contrast, detailed reports of cocaine psychoses are surprisingly rare. The first documented case is said to be that of Freud's friend Fleischl, although the effects described by Freud resemble toxic delirium more than classic stimulant psychosis (i.e., "white snakes crawling over his skin"; see Jones, 1953, p. 91).

The American medical literature dating from the time before cocaine was regulated contains only a few specific case descriptions of cocaine psychosis (although frequently there are generalized observations from clinical experience). The most specific description of a psychosis from this period is that of Norris (1901, p. 304):

> For several months he had been troubled with hallucinations of hearing and while semiconscious of his true condition, had avoided street cars and public gatherings where he imagined voices accused him of being a "cocaine fiend," etc. At night he would wander from room to room in his efforts to escape the voices which he heard talking about him, calling out, "Look he's going to take another"; and while reasoning with himself on the subjective character of his troubles, yet was impelled by their vividness to flee from them.

Gordon (1908, p. 99) gave an overall clinical characterization of 10 cases of "chronic intoxication" that he saw in which he emphasized "restlessness." Hallucinations of "sight, hearing and touch," particularly the feeling that "the skin is filled with insects, microbes, crystals of cocaine" and "delusive ideas which are mostly of a persecutory nature." Gordon also cited one specific case history of "a young physician" with "a systematized persecutory delusion concerning his mother and two brothers who conspired against him. Later he included another physician and myself in his delusive idea. The latter was intensified by terrifying hallucinations. He attempted to kill his mother on two occasions."

Owens (1912), based on experiences with 23 patients addicted to (but not necessarily psychotic from) cocaine, indicated that "hallucinations were not infrequently marked, including those of sight and common sensation associated with delusions of persecution, of suspicion and jealousy." He cited a case in which a woman injured herself because of "cocaine bugs," and another case in which psy-

chosis developed after a 4 gm dose: "Visual and auditory hallucinations with delusions of persecution occurred in a habitué who stated
he had snuffed 65 grains of cocaine. When apprehended this patient
was in the act of procuring his rifle to protect himself from imagin-
ary enemies."

Perhaps the most detailed account of cocaine psychosis published
to date is that of a patient of the neurologist Wilson (1940, p. 716),
previously cited by both Post (1976, p. 210) and Woods and Downs
(1973, p. 126).

> I imagined everyone was looking at me and watching me; even when locked in
> my room I could not persuade myself there were not watchers outside, with eyes
> glued to imaginary peepholes. If I ventured into the street I thought I was followed
> and that the passers-by made remarks about me; I thought my vice was known to
> all, and on all sides could hear the whispered word "Cocaine!" . . . It is curious
> that directly the effect of the cocaine has passed away all the suspicions and delu-
> sions vanish instantly. I could now see the absurdity and impossibility of the idea
> that a whole town was watching and talking about one obscure and unknown
> individual. I realized the folly of thinking that spies were in the room above,
> watching me through holes pierced in the ceiling. Yet the overpowering desire to
> repeat the dose would overtake me, and almost instantly after taking it all these
> delusions would return in full force, and no reasoning would banish them.

It is quite possible that this cursory review of the literature has
missed some cases of cocaine psychosis, and other cases are likely to
exist in the non-English literature. Nonetheless only four descriptions of specific patients were found in the American literature, and
this reviewer added a single case of manic psychosis after cocaine
(Angrist, 1983). It appears that cocaine psychosis may be more rare
than was previously assumed.

Other investigators have confirmed this view. Post (1976) noted
that Byck, after conducting a survey at a cocaine symposium, indicated that "few current workers in the field have seen a substantial
number of cases of cocaine psychosis." Resnick and Schuyten-Resnick (1976, p. 221) reviewed the literature on cocaine psychosis and
observed with some skepticism: "In searching for the scientific basis
for assertions regarding cocaine-induced psychosis, we found that
the reports in the medical literature are anecdotal and usually limited to the self-reports of a few individuals. There is a striking ab-
sence of information on the individuals' pre-morbid personality or
the circumstances or set in which the drug is taken." Nonetheless

they also cited as evidence in support of the concept of cocaine psychosis an experiment that was recorded on film (Isbell, 1953). In this study (Resnick & Schuyten-Resnick, 1976, p. 222) "a subject was given repeated intravenous injections of cocaine at short intervals beginning with 20 mg. every 30 min. and increasing to 50 mg. at 5 to 10 min. intervals. Over a 12-hour period, he received more than 2,000 mg. of cocaine at which time he began to show evidence of visual hallucinations (seeing insects) and had delusions that consisted of thoughts that he was being watched by detectives." Based on this and on more recent evidence Resnick and Schuyten-Resnick (personal communication) now acknowledge that cocaine can indeed frequently cause psychosis if high doses are taken.

This experiment was the first in which cocaine psychosis was induced prospectively under experimental conditions. More recently, Sherer et al. (1988) reported studies in which an IV bolus of cocaine was followed by an IV infusion calculated to maintain the high initial cocaine plasma level for several hours. Euphoria was found to diminish rapidly and anxiety and suspiciousness to emerge progressively. Overt paranoia was seen in three out of six subjects within four hours. Finally, Wesson and Smith (1985, p. 198) have indicated "a substantial increase in cocaine psychosis at the Haight Ashbury Free Medical Clinic due to the abuse of cocaine freebase." In discussing these psychoses Wesson and Smith stressed both that they occur in the context of high dose ("1 to 4 grams a day") and that they tend to be qualitatively "similar to the amphetamine psychosis but shorter in duration."

These data suggest that high dose and/or sustained plasma levels may be a sine qua non for the development of cocaine psychosis. The short half-life of cocaine, one hour or less (Javaid et al., 1978; Van Dyke & Byck, 1982), may make sustained plasma levels unlikely under "usual" conditions of abuse, thereby explaining the rarity of cocaine psychosis observed by investigators.

Amphetamine, on the other hand, has a much longer plasma half-life (10 to over 20 hours, depending on urine pH) (Beckett et al., 1965; Ebert et al., 1976; Kreuz & Axelrod, 1974). A half-life of this magnitude would make sustained plasma levels difficult to avoid even if a single large dose was taken, and would thereby predispose the user to the development of psychosis. Indeed, Kalant (1973) has documented 30 cases of psychosis with acute and subacute amphetamine intoxication, most of which occurred after single doses.

Thus, although amphetamine and cocaine are both capable of inducing psychosis, this seems to occur more frequently with amphetamine. Studies suggest that this difference may relate to differences in the half-lives of the two drugs. If so, these observations should have important implications for understanding the pathogenesis of CNS stimulant psychoses.

REFERENCES

Abelson, H. I. & Miller, J. D. (1985) A decade of trends in cocaine use in the household population. In: Kozel, N. J. & Adams, E. H. (Eds.), Cocaine use in America: Epidemiologic and clinical perspectives. NIDA Research Monograph 61, DHHS pub. no. (ADM) 85-1414. Washington, D.C.: Government Printing Office, 35–49.

Aldrich, M. R. & Barker, R. W. (1976) Historical aspects of cocaine use and abuse. In: Mule, S. J. (Ed.), Cocaine: Chemical, biological, clinical, social and treatment aspects. Cleveland: CRC Press, 3–11.

Angrist, B. (1983) Psychoses induced by central nervous system stimulants and related drugs. In: Creese, I. (Ed.), Stimulants: Neurochemical, behavioral and clinical perspectives. New York: Raven Press, 1–30.

Angrist, B. & Gershon, S. (1970) The phenomenology of experimentally induced amphetamine psychosis—preliminary observations. Biol. Psychiat. 2:95–107.

Angrist, B., Shopsin, B. & Gershon, S. (1972) Metabolites of monoamines in urine and cerebrospinal fluid after large dose amphetamine administration. Psychopharmacol. 26:1–9.

Angrist, B. & Sudilovsky, A. (1978) Central nervous system stimulants: Historical aspects and clinical effects. In: Iversen, L. L., Iversen, S. D. & Snyder, S. H. (Eds.), Handbook of psychopharmacology. Vol. 2: Stimulants. New York: Plenum Press, 99–165.

Beckett, A. H., Rowland, M. & Turner, P. (1965) Influence of urinary pH on excretion of amphetamine. Lancet 1:303.

Bell, D. S. (1973) The experimental reproduction of amphetamine psychosis. Arch. Gen. Psychiatr. 29:35–40.

Berg, D. F. (1970) Illicit use of dangerous drugs in the United States: A compilation of studies, surveys, and polls. Office of Science and Drug Abuse Prevention, Bureau of Narcotics and Dangerous Drugs, U.S. Dept. of Justice. Washington, D.C.: Government Printing Office.

Bett, W. R. (1946) Benzedrine sulfate in clinical medicine: A survey of the literature. Postgrad. Med. J. 22:205–218.

Brill, H. & Hirose, T. (1969) The rise and fall of a methamphetamine epidemic: Japan 1945–55. Sem. Psychiat. 1: 179–192.

Briscoe, O. V. & Hinterberger, H. (1968) A survey of the usage of amphetamines in parts of the Sydney community. *Med. J. Australia* 1:480–485.

Byck, R. (Ed.) (1974) *Cocaine papers by Sigmund Freud*. New York: Stonehill.

Clayton, R. J. (1985) Cocaine use in the United States: In a blizzard or just being snowed? In: Kozel, N. J. & Adams, E. H. (Eds.), *Cocaine use in America: Epidemiologic and clinical perspectives*. NIDA Research Monograph 61, DHHS pub. no. (ADM) 85-1414. Washington, D.C.: Government Printing Office, 8–34.

Connell, P. H. (1958). *Amphetamine psychosis*. Maudsley Monographs, no. 5. London: Oxford University Press.

Ebert, M. H., van Kammen, D. P. & Murphy, D. C. (1976) Plasma levels of amphetamine and behavioral response. In: Gottschalk, L. & Merlis, S. (Eds.), *Pharmacokinetics of psychoactive drugs, blood levels and clinical response*. New York: Spectrum Publications, 157–169.

Editorial. (1885) *Lancet* 2:123.

Erickson, P. G., Adlaf, E. M., Murray, G. S. & Smart, R. G. (1987) *The steel drug cocaine in perspective*. Lexington, Mass.: Lexington Books, D.C. Heath, 58.

Gallup Organization. (1969) *Newsweek*, Dec. 29, 42–45.

Gawin, F. H. (1986) New uses of antidepressants in cocaine abuse. *Psychosomatics* 27(Suppl. 11):24–29.

Gawin, F. H. & Kleber, H. D. (1985) Cocaine use in a treatment population: Patterns and diagnostic distinctions. In: Kozel, N. J. & Adams, E. H. (Eds.), *Cocaine use in America: Epidemiologic and clinical perspectives*. NIDA Research Monograph 61, DHHS pub. no. (ADM) 85-1414. Washington, D.C.: Government Printing Office, 182–192.

Gold, M. S., Washton, A. M. & Dackis, C. A. (1985) Cocaine abuse:

Neurochemistry, phenomenology, and treatment. In: Kozel, N. J. & Adams, E. H. (Eds.), *Cocaine use in America*, 130–155.

Gordon, A. (1908) Insanities caused by acute and chronic intoxications with opium and cocaine. *JAMA* 51:97–101.

Greenberg, J. R. & Lustig, N. (1966) Misuse of the Dristan inhaler. *NY State J. Med.* 66:613–617.

Griffith, J. (1966) A study of illicit amphetamine drug traffic in Oklahoma City. *Am. J. Psychiat.* 123:560–569.

Griffith, J., Cavanaugh, J., Held, J. & Oates, J. (1972) Dextroamphetamine evaluation of psychotomimetic properties in man. *Arch. Gen. Psychiat.* 26:97–100.

Griffith, J., Davis, J. & Oates, J. (1971) Amphetamines: Addiction to a non-addicting drug. *Pharmakopsychiatrie Neuro-Psychopharmacologie* 4:58–64.

Griffith, J., Oates, J. & Cavanaugh, J. (1968) Paranoid episodes induced by drug. *JAMA* 205:39, 46.

Grinspoon, L. & Hedblom, P. (1975) *The speed culture*. Cambridge, Mass.: Harvard University Press.

Guttman, E. & Sargeant, W. (1937) Observations on Benzedrine. *Br. Med. J.* 1:1013–1015.

Hemmi, T. (1969) How we handled the problem of drug abuse in Japan. In: Sjoqvist, F. & Tottie, M. (Eds.), *Abuse of central stimulants*. Stockholm: Almqvist and Wiskell, 147–153.

Inghe, G. (1969) The present state of abuse and addiction to stimulant drugs in Sweden. In: Sjoqvist, F. & Tottie, M. (Eds.), *Abuse of central stimulants*. Stockholm: Almqvist and Wiskell, 187–214.

Isbell, H. (1953) *Clinical manifestations of drug addiction* (Film). Made at the Addiction Research Center, Lexington, Kentucky.

Javaid, J. I., Fischman, M. W., Schuster, C. R., Dekermenjian, H. & Davis, J. M. (1978) Cocaine plasma concentration: Relation to physiological and subjective effects in humans. *Science* 202:227–228.

Jekel, J. F., Podlewski, H., Dean-Patterson, S., Allen, D. F., Clarke, N. & Cartwright, P. (1986) Epidemic free-base cocaine abuse case study from the Bahamas. *Lancet* 1:459–462.

Jeri, F. R. (1984) Coca-paste smoking in some Latin America countries: A review of a severe and unabated form of addiction. *Bull. Narc.* 36:15–32.

Jones, E. (1953) *The life and works of Sigmund Freud*, vol. 1 (1856–1900). New York: Basic Books, 78–97.

Kalant, O. J. (1973) *The amphetamines: Toxicity and addiction*. Brookside Monographs of the Addiction Research Foundation, no. 5. Toronto: University of Toronto Press.

Kiloh, L. G. & Brandon, S. (1962) Habituation and addiction to amphetamines. *Br. Med. J.* 2:40–43.

Kramer, J. C., Fischmann, V. S. & Littlefield, D. C. (1967) Amphetamine abuse: Pattern and effects of high doses taken intravenously. *JAMA* 201:305–309.

Kreuz, D. S. & Axelrod, J. (1974) Amphetamine in human plasma: A sensitive and specific enzymatic assay. *Science* 183:420–421.

Lesses, M. F. & Myerson, A. (1938) Benzedrine sulfate. *JAMA* 110:1507–1508.

Masaki, T. (1956) The amphetamine problem in Japan. *World Health Organ. Tech. Rep. Serv.* 102:14–21.

Mattison, J. B. (1891) Cocaine poisoning. *Med. and Surg. Reporter* 65:645–650.

McConnell, W. B. (1963) Amphetamine substances in mental illnesses in Northern Ireland. *Br. J. Psychiat.* 109:218–224.

McNeil, D. (1967) An amphetamine apple in psychedelic eden. *Village Voice*, February 2, pp. 11 and 31.

Meyers, A. C. (1902) *Eight years in cocaine hell*. Chicago: Press of the St. Luke Society.

Monroe, R. R. & Drell, H. J. (1947) Oral use of stimulants obtained from inhalers. *JAMA* 135:909–915.

Norris, G. W. (1901) A case of cocaine habit of ten month's duration treated by complete and immediate withdrawal of the drug. *Philadelphia Med. J.* 7:304–305.

O'Malley, P. M., Johnston, L. D. & Bachman, J. D. (1985) Cocaine use among American adolescents and young adults. In: Kozel, N. J. & Adams, E. H. (Eds.), *Cocaine use in America: Epidemiologic and clinical perspectives*. NIDA Research Monograph 61, DHHS pub. no. (ADM) 85-1414. Washington, D.C.: Government Printing Office, 50–75.

Owens, W. D. (1912) Signs and symptoms presented by those addicted to cocaine. *JAMA* 58:329–330.

Peterson, R. C. (1977) History of cocaine. In: Peterson, R. C. & Stillman, R. C. (Eds.), *Cocaine, 1977*. NIDA Research Monograph 13, DHHS pub. no. (ADM) 77-432. Washington, D.C.: Government Printing Office, 17–34.

Post, R. M. (1976) Clinical aspects of cocaine: Assessment of acute chronic effects in animals and man. In: Mule, S. J. (Ed.), *Cocaine: Chemical, biological, clinical, social and treatment aspects*. Cleveland: CRC Press, 203–215.

Prinzmetal, M. & Bloomberg, W. (1935) Use of Benzedrine for the treatment of narcolepsy. *JAMA* 105:2051–2054.

Reifenstein, E. C., Jr. & Davidoff, E. (1939) Benzedrine sulfate therapy, the present status. *NY State J. Med.* 39: 42–57.

Resnick, R. B. & Schuyten-Resnick, E. (1976) Clinical aspects of cocaine: Assessment of cocaine abuse behavior in man. In: Mule, S. J. (Ed.), *Cocaine: Chemical, biological, clinical, social and treatment aspects.* Cleveland: CRC Press, 219–228.

Rylander, G. (1969) Clinical and medico-criminological aspects of addiction to central stimulating drugs. In: Sjoqvist, F. & Tottie, M. (Eds.), *Abuse of central stimulants.* Stockholm: Almqvist and Wiskell, 251–273.

Sadusk, J. R. (1966) Non-narcotic addiction: Size and extent of the problem. *JAMA* 196:707–709.

Schultz, M. G. (1971) The "strange case" of Robert Louis Stevenson. *JAMA* 216:90–94.

Sherer, M., Kumor, K., Cone, E. & Jaffe, J. H. (1988) Suspiciousness induced by four-hour intravenous infusions of cocaine. *Arch. Gen. Psychiat.* 45:673–677.

Siegel, R. K. (1979) Cocaine smoking. *N. Engl. J. Med.* 300:373.

Siegel, R. K. (1985) New patterns of cocaine use: Changing doses and routes. In: Kozel, N. J. & Adams, E. H. (Eds.), *Cocaine use in America: Epidemiologic and clinical perspectives.* NIDA Research Monograph 61, DHHS pub. no. (ADM) 85-1414. Washington, D.C.: Government Printing Office, 204–220.

Smith, R. (1969) The world of the Haight-Ashbury speed freak. *J. Psychedel. Drugs* 2:172–188.

Snyder, S. H. (1974) *Madness and the brain.* New York: McGraw-Hill.

Time magazine. (1937) May 10, 45.

Van Dyke, C. & Byck, R. (1982) Cocaine. *Sci. Am.* 246:128–141.

Vondracek, V., Prokupek, J., Fischer, R. & Ahrenbergova, M. (1968) Recent patterns of addiction in Czechoslovakia. *Br. J. Psychiat* 114:285–292.

Waud, S. P. (1938) The effects of toxic doses of benzyl methyl carbinamine (Benzedrine) in man. *JAMA* 110:206–207.

Wesson, D. R. & Smith, D. E. (1985) Cocaine: Treatment perspectives. In: Kozel, N. J. & Adams, E. H. (Eds.), *Cocaine use in America: Epidemiologic and clinical perspectives.* NIDA Research Monograph 61, DHHS pub. no. (ADM) 85-1414. Washington, D.C.: Government Printing Office, 193–203.

Wilson, S.A.K. (1940) *Neurology* (edited by Bruce, A. N.), vol. 1. Baltimore: Williams and Wilkins, 716.

Woods, J. H. & Downs, D. A. (1973) The psychopharmacology of cocaine. In: *Drug use in America: Problem in perspective.* Appendix. The technical papers of the National Commission on Marijuana and Drug Abuse. Vol. 1: *Patterns and consequences of drug use.* Washington, D.C.: Government Printing Office.

Young, D. & Scoville, W. B. (1938) Paranoid psychosis in narcolepsy and the possible danger of Benzedrine treatment. *Med. Clin. N. Am.* 22:637–646.

2

Populations at Risk
for Cocaine Use and Subsequent
Consequences

*Edgar H. Adams, Beatrice A. Rouse, and
Joseph C. Gfroerer*

Although by 1972 14% of youth aged 12–17 and 48% of young adults aged 18–25 had tried marijuana, the prevalence of lifetime cocaine use was only 1.5% and 9%, respectively. Since that time, dramatic increases in the prevalence of cocaine use have been noted and cocaine use has been labeled a major public health problem (Adams & Durell, 1984).

The number of people trying cocaine at least once (lifetime prevalence) increased from 5.4 million in 1974 to 22.2 million in 1985. The estimated number of "current" users (use in the past 30 days) of cocaine increased from 1.6 million in 1977 to 4.3 million in 1979, remained stable at about 4.2 million in 1982, and increased to 5.8 million in 1985 (Kozel & Adams, 1986). The increase in current users between 1982 and 1985 occurred while use in the previous year remained relatively stable at approximately 12 million.

Subsequent to the dramatic increases in cocaine use in the late 1970s and early 1980s, increases in emergency room episodes and treatment admissions were also noted. These increases have been cited as evidence that the incidence of cocaine use is also increasing. On the other hand, others have noted that increases in emergencies and entries into treatment reflect other factors such as use of drugs in combination, changing routes of administration, and in the case of treatment admissions, the lag time between first use and treatment (Adams & Kozel, 1985).

In 1984 and 1985, questions on cocaine use were added to several waves of the Gallup poll. These data suggest a small increase in use (among males) but no indication of the dramatic rise in prevalence suggested in the press (Adams et al., 1985).

However, data from the 1985 Gallup poll survey of high school seniors indicated that current use of cocaine increased for the second year in a row. At least a portion of the increase could probably be attributed to "crack," a form of freebase that was sold in a unit dose amount for under $25. With cocaine available at this price, the price barrier previously thought to limit use among students was effectively removed. Although the 1986 high school senior data indicated a plateauing of current use at 6.2%, there is still concern about the use of crack by our young people. Of the 1985 high school seniors who reported using cocaine in the past year, one-third used crack. Similarly, among youth aged 12–17, 44% of those who tried cocaine had smoked it.

The use of "crack," which is normally smoked, has increased concerns about more rapid addiction and severe consequences associated with its use. However, the continued danger of intranasal use cannot be overlooked.

In 1984 and 1985, a number of cases of myocardial infarction in intranasal cocaine users were reported in the literature (Cregler & Mark, 1985; Howard et al., 1985; Pasternack et al., 1985; Schachne et al., 1984). Other studies reported such symptoms as depression, anxiety, irritability, apathy, and paranoia in a large proportion of cases (Chitwood, 1985). Although it has been suggested that IV use and freebasing or smoking of cocaine often lead to increased frequency of use, escalation of dosage, and rapid development of severe dependence, a study of Gawin and Kleber noted that intranasal users had a higher proportion of subjects with axis 1 diagnosis than other users, thus suggesting that dangers associated with the intranasal administration of cocaine have been underestimated (Gawin & Kleber, 1985; Van Dyke & Byck, 1982). Others have also noted that freebase cocaine users were no more likely than intranasal or intravenous users to have experienced psychotic symptoms, withdrawal effects, or tolerance (Brower et al., 1986).

The increases in prevalence of cocaine use, coupled with increasing treatment admissions and emergency room cases, raise a number of questions concerning the population at risk for cocaine use, the use of other drugs in combination with cocaine, the progression of cocaine use, and the dependency associated with it.

POPULATION AT RISK OF COCAINE USE

Although the reputation of cocaine has been that of a chic drug used by the wealthy, analysis of preliminary data from the 1985 National Household Survey on Drug Abuse indicates that cocaine use is well distributed throughout our population among all income groups (Tables 2.1, 2.2). Cocaine use is found among the employed and unemployed segments of our population, although it is greater among the unemployed. It is interesting to note that use among homemakers and those who are married is lower than among other groups. The highest prevalence is found among those who are co-habiting. As is the case with most illicit drug use prevalence is higher among males. Lifetime prevalence is higher among white

TABLE 2.1

Cocaine Use by Demographic and Other Characteristics, 1985 (Preliminary File)

Subgroup	% Ever used		% Used in past month	
	Youth 12–17	Adults 18–44	Youth 12–17	Adults 18–44
Total	4.9	18.6	★	4.9
Sex				
Male	5.8	22.8		6.2
Female	3.9	14.5		3.7
Race				
White	5.2	20.6		5.1
Black	2.3	13.6		5.0
Hispanic	6.7	9.8		3.2
Region				
Northeast	6.1	18.8		5.3
North Central	3.2	16.5		3.8
South	2.6	16.0		2.6
West	8.8	25.0		8.6
Population density				
Large metro	5.6	22.6		6.8
Small metro	5.7	19.3		4.7
Nonmetro	3.5	15.6		4.2

SOURCE: NIDA, National Survey on Drug Abuse, 1985.
★*N* is too small to report

TABLE 2.2

Cocaine Use by Socioeconomic Characteristics among Adults 18–44
(Preliminary File)

	% Ever used	% Used in past month
Personal income		
<$5,000	18.5	6.1
5,000–8,999	19.6	5.1
9,000–14,999	20.3	5.6
15,000–19,999	20.5	4.3
20,000–29,999	21.2	5.9
30,000–50,000	19.2	2.8
>50,000	15.3	3.8
Employment		
Working full-time	19.7	5.0
Working part-time	16.1	3.6
Unemployed	24.0	8.0
Homemaker	10.7	3.8
Student	17.0	3.3
Marital status		
Married	13.1	2.4
Divorced/separated	24.4	4.9
Cohabiting	41.7	14.0
Never married	25.4	9.1

SOURCE: NIDA, National Survey on Drug Abuse, 1985.

adults than among black or Hispanic adults. In contrast, among youth, Hispanics have the higher prevalence. The prevalence of cocaine use is higher in the northeastern and western than in the north central and southern regions of the country, and it is also greater in metropolitan areas.

A study of cocaine users aged 26+ years between 1979 and 1982 indicated an increase in use in this age group in 1982. This increase continued in 1985. In an initial attempt to look further at the demographics of new cocaine users, a population was identified from the 1982 National Survey on Drug Abuse who first used cocaine after age 25 and in the period between 1979 and 1982. These new users were more likely to be unmarried, employed, college graduates, residing in metropolitan areas, and in the western part of the

United States (Table 2.3). The lack of significant sex differences suggests the possibility of an increased willingness to experiment with drugs by women. Although a population of new cocaine users aged 26 and older was identified, there were relatively few new users of marijuana in this age group. This suggests that the age of risk for initiation of use may be longer for cocaine than for other drugs (Adams et al., 1986; Kandel et al., 1985; O'Malley et al., 1985; Raveis & Kandel, 1987).

The present emphasis on the phenomenon of cocaine use has drawn attention to the cocaine user as having a single drug problem. However, in general, cocaine users have already experienced the use of other drugs, especially marijuana. Only 4% of cocaine users have either never used marijuana or used cocaine at an earlier age (Table 2.4). Furthermore, the probability of cocaine use increases with the frequency of marijuana use (Table 2.5). More than 70% of those who used marijuana 200 or more times in their lifetime also used cocaine, versus less than 0.5% of those who never used marijuana. A similar relationship was demonstrated in the mid-seventies. In this study 82% of those using marijuana 1,000 or more times had tried cocaine compared to 77% of those using marijuana 200 or more times (Clayton & Voss, 1981). This change

TABLE 2.3

Demographic Characteristics of New Cocaine Users Aged 26 and Older (First Use within Past 3 Years and after Age 25)

Demographics	New cocaine users	All 25–50-year-olds	t-test
	(N = 82)	(N = 2,102)	(5% sig. level)
% White	86	79	NS
% Male	53	48	NS
% West region	38	21	S
% Metro area	95	79	S
% Not married	65	35	S
% College graduate	44	26	S
% Employed	91	76	S
% Manager or professional	61	35	S
% Income ≥$30,000	34	31	NS

SOURCE: NIDA, National Survey on Drug Abuse, 1985.

TABLE 2.4

Sequence of Use of Marijuana among Lifetime Cocaine Users (Persons Who Have Used Cocaine at Least Once)

	% Distribution
Never used marijuana	8
Used cocaine, then later marijuana	2
First used cocaine and marijuana at same age	8
Used marijuana, then later cocaine	88

Source: NIDA, National Survey on Drug Abuse, 1985.

probably reflects the large increase in the number of cocaine users that has occurred since the mid-seventies. Previous research has also demonstrated a relationship between cocaine use and the recency of marijuana use (Adams et al., 1986).

The analysis of new cocaine users aged 26 and older based on 1982 data also demonstrates the relationship between cocaine use and the frequency of marijuana use. Compared to a group of 26- to 50-year-olds who had used marijuana but not cocaine, new cocaine users were more likely to have used marijuana in the past month and to have used it at least 100 times (Table 2.6).

In an attempt to examine the extent to which marijuana use pre-

TABLE 2.5

Cocaine Use among Adults Aged 18 and Over by Lifetime Frequency of Marijuana Use

Frequency of marijuana use	% Ever used cocaine	% Never used cocaine
Never	0.3	99.7
1–2 times	6.0	94.0
3–5 times	10.4	89.6
6–10 times	18.8	81.2
11–49 times	32.3	67.7
50–99 times	50.3	49.7
100–199 times	58.9	41.1
200+ times	77.3	22.7

Source: NIDA, National Survey on Drug Abuse, 1985.

TABLE 2.6
Drug Use of New Cocaine Users Aged 26 and Older (First Use within Past 3 Years and after Age 25)

	New cocaine users	All 26–50-year-olds who have used marijuana but not cocaine	t-test
	(N = 82)	(N = 628)	(5% sig. level)
Cocaine use			
% Past month	21	0	—
% Past year	57	0	—
Marijuana use			
% Past month	51	14	S
% Past year	74	29	S
% Ever	96	100	NS
% At least 100 times	53	14	S
% First use before age 18	22	21	NS

SOURCE: NIDA, National Survey on Drug Abuse, 1985.

dicts cocaine use, regression analysis was performed using any lifetime use of cocaine as the dependent variable. After controlling for age, race, and sex, the number of times marijuana was used in a lifetime was the strongest predictor. The adjusted R^2 for this model was .43. Thus, the population at greatest risk for cocaine use is more likely to consist of current and frequent users of marijuana.

MULTIPLE DRUG USE

The use of marijuana is important not only as an antecedent variable with regard to initiating cocaine use, but because it is often used in conjunction with cocaine. In a National Institute on Drug Abuse (NIDA)-sponsored study, questions were added to the Gallup poll in 1984 and 1985. The resulting data indicating that cocaine users not only used other drugs but often used them in combination with cocaine. In many cases, these drugs were taken to modify the crash associated with cocaine use. Half the cocaine users indicated

that they took alcohol and cocaine together and 35% used marijuana when using cocaine.

These data on combined drug use are supported by data on treatment admissions (from 15 states), which indicate that in 1984 cocaine was reported as either a primary or secondary problem in
almost 20% of all admissions to treatment. In cases where cocaine
was reported as the primary drug of abuse, a secondary drug problem was reported in almost 80% of cases. The drugs most often
reported as being used in combination with cocaine are marijuana,
alcohol, and heroin. Data from cases reported by emergency rooms
in 1985 reflect a similar pattern. Slightly more than 60% of the cases
reflect cocaine use in combination. Again, the most frequently mentioned combinations are cocaine and heroin, alcohol and cocaine,
and cocaine and marijuana. One implication of this is that patients
seeking treatment for cocaine use may in fact be dually addicted and
therefore present a more complex treatment problem that might
otherwise be anticipated. For example, in one study more than 30%
of cocaine patients also have had a DSM-III diagnosis of alcohol
abuse (Gawin & Kleber, 1985).

PROGRESSION OF COCAINE USE

As has been noted, those who currently and frequently use marijuana are more likely to use cocaine, but the question remains
whether a cocaine user will progress to more intensive and destructive patterns of cocaine use. Van Dyke and Byck have suggested
that the smoking or injection of cocaine can lead to almost continuous consumption and drug-seeking behavior, destructive to personal competence and productivity (Van Dyke & Byck, 1982).
Gawin and Kleber noted that freebase smokers used twice as much
cocaine weekly as other groups (Gawin & Kleber, 1985). Analysis
of treatment data suggests that the IV or freebase user is more likely
to be a frequent user than the intranasal cocaine user. Analyzing
data based on a follow-up of high school seniors, and using an in-
dex based on frequency of use, O'Malley and his colleagues have
addressed the issue of progression (Table 2.7) (O'Malley et al.,
1985). The analysis indicated that three to four years after gradua-
tion, 4.7% of the population had used cocaine 10 or more times in

TABLE 2.7
Longitudinal Patterns of Annual Use of Cocaine: Classes of 1976–1980

Base-year use	First follow-up use	Second follow-up use
92.18% (none)	84.12% (none)	75.39% (none)
		7.59% (<ten)
		1.14% (ten+)
	6.85% (<ten)	2.33% (none)
		3.46% (<ten)
		1.06% (ten+)
	1.23% (ten+)	0.20% (none)
		0.55% (<ten)
		0.48% (ten+)
6.63% (ten)	2.14% (none)	1.25% (none)
		0.71% (<ten)
		0.18% (ten+)
	3.35% (<ten)	0.81% (none)
		1.79% (<ten)
		0.75% (ten+)
	1.13% (ten+)	0.09% (none)
		0.38% (<ten)
		0.67% (ten+)
1.20% (ten+)	0.28% (none)	0.20% (none)
		0.08% (<ten)
		0.01% (ten+)
	0.38% (<ten)	0.05% (none)
		0.21% (<ten)
		0.13% (ten+)
	0.52% (ten+)	0.03% (none)
		0.22% (<ten)
		0.27% (ten+)

SOURCE: O'Malley et al. (1985).
NOTE: Data are based on approximately 7,000 respondents who participated in two follow-ups.
Entries sum up to 100% within each column.

the previous year compared to only 1.2% of the respective graduating classes. Also interesting to note is the transition between levels of use. It would seem, then, that although progression to increased levels of use may occur, it is not inevitable.

DEPENDENCY MEASURES

The issue of progression is an important one because of the current belief that cocaine is a powerfully addictive drug and that consequences associated with its use will continue to increase unless the using population diminishes in size or reduces its level of use. In the past, cocaine was not considered addictive because the definition of addiction was based on the opiate model in which physical dependence manifested by serious withdrawal symptoms was required for a drug to be considered addictive.

The *Diagnostic and Statistical Manual of Mental Disorders* (third edition) (DSM-III) classifies substance use disorders as either substance abuse or substance dependence. *Substance abuse* is defined as comprising (a) a pattern of pathological use, (b) impairment in social or occupational functioning due to substance use and (c) minimal duration of disturbance of at least one month. Abuse differs from dependence in that a diagnosis of dependence requires the presence of tolerance or withdrawal. Because it was thought that only transitory withdrawal symptoms occurred after cessation or reduction of cocaine, the DSM-III contains no cocaine dependence category.

Recent revisions to the criteria for psychoactive substance use disorders included in the DSM-III(R) contain categories for cocaine abuse and cocaine dependence. Psychoactive *substance dependence* is defined as follows:

A. At least three of the following:
  1. Substance often taken in larger amounts over a longer period than the individual intended
  2. Persistent desire or one or more unsuccessful efforts to cut down or control substance use
  3. A great deal of time spent in activities necessary to get the substance, take the substance, or recover from its effects
  4. Frequent intoxication or withdrawal symptoms when expected to fulfill major role obligations or when substance use is physically hazardous

5. Important social, occupational, or recreational activities given up or reduced because of substance use
6. Continued substance use despite knowledge of having a persistent or recurrent social, occupational, psychological, or physical problem that is caused or exacerbated by the use of the substance
7. Marked tolerance: Need for markedly increased amounts of the substance in order to achieve intoxication or desired effect, or markedly diminished effect with continued use of the same amount
8. Characteristic withdrawal symptoms
9. Substance often taken to relieve or avoid withdrawal symptoms.

B. Some symptoms of the disturbance have persisted for at least one month, or have occurred repeatedly over a longer period of time. Thus, a diagram of dependence no longer requires tolerance and withdrawal.

Furthermore, in the popular concept of addiction compulsive use or loss of control has been recognized as a key determinant. It is by applying this criterion that cocaine is now being labeled "addicting."

Animal studies have shown that cocaine functions as a positive reinforcer, that is, it maintains responding behavior in animals (Johanson, 1984). In fact, cocaine is such a powerful reinforcing drug that many researchers use cocaine to train animals to self-administer drugs. In an experiment in which laboratory rats were given unlimited access to intravenous cocaine or heroin, Bozarth and Wise demonstrated that animals allowed access to heroin demonstrated patterns of stable self-administration of the drug (Bozarth & Wise, 1985). In contrast, animals self-administering cocaine rapidly developed patterns of episodic drug intake with periods of excessive cocaine self-administration. At the end of 30 days of testing, 36% of the animals self-administering heroin and 90% of those self-administering cocaine were dead. This study, as well as earlier studies, demonstrates that animals, given unlimited access to cocaine, will engage in compulsive, uncontrolled patterns of cocaine use to the point of death (Johanson et al., 1976). Finally, in a breaking point study with cocaine, large primates pressed a lever up to 12 thousand times to get one small infusion of cocaine (Yanagita, 1973).

Smoking cocaine freebase, then, may lead to loss of control

manifested by an almost continuous consumption and drug-seeking behavior destructive to personal competence and productivity. Analysis of emergency room and treatment data suggests that in these populations of individuals suffering consequences associated with cocaine use, shifts to IV use and freebasing were in fact occurring. For example, in 1977, emergency room data showed that less than 1% of cases were associated with smoking or freebasing of cocaine. By 1984, 6% of emergency room cases were associated with cocaine smoking, and by the second half of 1986, 25% of all cocaine cases reported smoking as the route of administration. Similar increases were noted in admissions to treatment facilities. In 1979, 1% of admissions for cocaine abuse reported that smoking was their primary route of administration. By 1984, this had risen to 19%.

Because of the increasing concern about dependency associated with cocaine, a self-reported dependency scale based on the Diagnostic Interview Schedule was included in the 1985 National Household Survey on Drug Abuse. The scale consisted of four questions that included whether the user ever felt tolerant to, or dependent on, a particular drug, suffered withdrawal symptoms, or tried to cut down on use. In a preliminary study, a sample of 100 high-risk cocaine users aged 20–40 was drawn from respondents to the Household Survey. A high-risk cocaine user was defined as one who had used cocaine at least 12 times during the past year.

A review of the sample indicated that 96 of the 100 cases also used marijuana. In fact, most were long-term marijuana users, with 87% having used marijuana for more than 6 years and 60% for more than 10 years (Table 2.8). In contrast, 53% of the sample had been using cocaine for less than 5 years. We also noted that the high-risk group was roughly two-thirds male, although interestingly, more recent users, that is, less than 4 years, were equally likely to be female.

Although more than half (56%) of the sample exhibited one or more symptoms from the dependency scale, there was a clear delineation by frequency of use (Table 2.9). Of the sample with usage levels of once a week or more, 75% reported one or more dependence symptoms versus only 40% of those with usage levels of once or twice a month. Some dependence or withdrawal symptoms were reported at all levels "trying to cut down" and "feeling effects" were reported most often (Table 2.10).

TABLE 2.8
Percent Distribution of Years since First Use for Marijuana and Cocaine in a Sample of Frequent Past-Year Cocaine Users Aged 20–40

Drug	Years since first use			
	2	3–5	6–9	10 +
Marijuana	4	9	27	60
Cocaine	23	30	23	24

SOURCE: NIDA, National Survey on Drug Abuse, 1985.

TABLE 2.9
Percent Distribution of the Number of Symptoms Reported in a Self-Reported Dependency Scale by Frequency of Use in the Past Year among a High-Risk Sample of Cocaine Users

Frequency of use	Number of symptoms				
	0	1	2	3	4
Once a week or more	25	42	21	4	8
3 times/month	36	33	24	6	0
1–2 times/month	60	28	12	12	0
Total	44	33	18	3	2

SOURCE: NIDA, National Survey on Drug Abuse, 1985.

TABLE 2.10
Percent Distribution of Symptoms Attributed to Cocaine in a Self-Reported Dependency Scale by Frequency of Use in the Past Year among a High-Risk Sample of Cocaine Users

Frequency of use	Tolerance	Dependence	Withdrawal	Cutdown
Once a week or more	42	13	13	63
3 times/month	36	9	9	45
1–2 times/month	19	5	2	26
Total	30	8	7	41

SOURCE: NIDA, National Survey on Drug Abuse, 1985.

TABLE 2.11
Percent Distribution of Routes of Administration
Ever Used among a High-Risk Sample of Cocaine
Users

Sniff only	40
Freebase only	6
IV only	2
Sniff + freebase	26
Sniff + IV	3
Other combinations	23

SOURCE: NIDA, National Survey on Drug Abuse, 1985.

The self-reported measures of cocaine dependency were also examined to determine any association with route of administration.
Forty percent of the high-risk sample reported sniffing as the only
route of administration (Table 2.11); approximately one-third of the
same sample reported that they had tried freebasing cocaine. A majority of the high-risk cocaine users (52%) had tried several routes
of administration.

Although the number of symptoms was distributed unequally
when looked at by route of administration, only 44% of the snor-
ters reported symptoms compared to 70% of those who said they
had tried freebasing (Table 2.12). As before, tolerance and attempts
to cut back were the most reported symptoms, with attempts to cut
back being highest among freebasers. It should also be noted that
dependence and withdrawal were reported more among users of

TABLE 2.12
Percent Distribution of the Number of Symptoms Reported in a Self-
Reported Dependency Scale by Route of Administration in the Past Year
among a High-Risk Sample of Cocaine Users

	Number of symptoms				
Route of administration	0	1	2	3	4
Sniff only	56	20	18	3	18
Freebase + others	30	45	25	0	0
Other combinations	42	33	0	17	8

SOURCE: NIDA, National Survey on Drug Abuse, 1985.

TABLE 2.13
Percent Distribution of Symptoms Attributed to Cocaine in a Self-
Reported Dependency Scale by Route of Administration in the Past Year
among a High-Risk Sample of Cocaine Users

Route of cocaine administration	Cocaine symptoms			
	Tolerance	Dependence	Withdrawal	Cutback
Sniff only	28	10	8	28
Freebase + others	34	5	2	55
Other combinations	33	17	25	42

Source: NIDA, National Survey on Drug Abuse, 1985.

other combinations, which include the intravenous route of administration (Table 2.13).

In summary, the cocaine user is likely to be a marijuana user,
with marijuana use preceding cocaine use. Furthermore, the probability of cocaine use increases both with the recency and frequency
of marijuana use. Seventy-seven percent of marijuana users who
have used marijuana 200 or more times have also tried cocaine,
versus less than 1% of those who have not tried cocaine. In addition, data from a variety of sources indicate that the cocaine user is
not only likely to be a polydrug user, but also likely to use cocaine
in combination with other drugs, such as alcohol, marijuana, and
heroin. This raises the possibility of dual dependence, which may
further complicate the treatment process. Data from a high-risk
sample of cocaine users suggest that symptoms attributed to cocaine
use on the self-reported dependency scale are present at all use levels
for all routes of administration, including the population that only
reports having snorted the drug. These preliminary results not only
suggest that dependency to cocaine can and does occur, they also
further dispel the myth that cocaine is a benign drug as long as it is
taken by the intranasal route of administration.

REFERENCES

Adams, E. H. & Durell, J. (1984)
Cocaine: A growing public health prob-
lem. In: Grabowski, J. (Ed.), *Cocaine:
Pharmacology, effects, and treatment of*
abuse. NIDA Research Monograph 50,
DHHS pub. no. (ADM) 84-1326.
Washington, D.C.: Government Print-
ing Office, 9–14.

Adams, E. H., Gfroerer, J. C. & Blanken, A. J. (1985) Prevalence, patterns and consequences of cocaine use. In: Brink, C. H. (Ed.), *Cocaine: A symposium*. Madison: Wisconsin Institute of Drug Abuse, 37–42.

Adams, E. H., Gfroerer, J. C., Rouse, B. A. & Kozel, N. J. (1986) Trends in prevalence and consequences of cocaine use. *Cocaine: Pharmacology, addiction, and therapy*, vol. 6, no. 2, Advances in Alcohol and Substance Abuse series.

Adams, E. H. & Kozel, N. J. (1985) Cocaine use in America: Introduction and overview. In: Kozel, N. J. & Adams, E. H. (Eds.), *Cocaine use in America: Epidemiologic and clinical perspectives*. NIDA Research Monograph 61, DHHS pub. no. (ADM) 85-1414. Washington, D.C.: Government Printing Office, 1–7.

Bozarth, M. A. & Wise, R. A. (1985) Toxicity associated with long-term intravenous heroin and cocaine self-administration in the rat. *JAMA* 254 (1):81–83.

Brower, K. J., Hierholzer, R. & Maddahian, U. (1986) Recent trends in cocaine abuse in a VA psychiatric population. *Hospit. Commun. Psychiat.* 37: 1229–1234.

Chitwood, D. D. (1985) Patterns and consequences of cocaine use. In: Kozel, N. J. & Adams, E. H. (Eds.), *Cocaine use in America: Epidemiologic and clinical perspectives*. NIDA Research Monograph 61, DHHS pub. no. (ADM) 85-1414. Washington, D.C.: Government Printing Office, 111–129.

Clayton, R. R. & Voss, H. L. (1981) Young men and drugs in Manhattan: A causal analysis. NIDA Research Monograph 39, DHHS pub. no. (ADM) 81-1167. Washington, D.C.: Government Printing Office.

Cregler, L. L. & Mark, H. (1985) Relation of acute myocardial infarction to cocaine abuse. *Am. J. Cardiol.* 56: 784.

Gawin, F. H. & Kleber, H. D. (1985) Cocaine use in a treatment population: Patterns and diagnostic distinctions. In: Kozel, N. J. & Adams, E. H. (Eds.), *Cocaine use in America: Epidemiologic and clinical perspectives*. NIDA Research Monograph 61, DHHS pub. no. (ADM) 85-1414. Washington, D.C.: Government Printing Office, 182–192.

Howard, R. E., Hueter, D. C. & Davis, G. J. (1985) Acute myocardial infarction following cocaine abuse in a young woman with normal coronary arteries. *JAMA* 254:95–96.

Johanson, C. E. (1984) Assessment of the dependence potential of cocaine in animals. In: Grabowski, J. (Ed.), *Cocaine: Pharmacology, effects, and treatment of abuse*. NIDA Research Monograph 50, DHHS pub. no. (ADM) 84-1326. Washington, D.C.: Government Printing Office, 54–71.

Johanson, C. E., Balster, R. L. & Bonese, K. (1976) Self-administration of psychomotor stimulant drugs: The effects of unlimited access. *Pharmacol. Biochem. Behav.* 4:45–51.

Kandel, D. B., Murphy, D. & Karus, D. (1985) Cocaine use in young adulthood: Patterns of use and psychosocial correlates. In: Kozel, N. J. & Adams, E. H. (Eds.), *Cocaine use in America: Epidemiologic and clinical perspectives*. NIDA Research Monograph 61, DHHS pub. no. (ADM) 85-1414. Washington, D.C.: Government Printing Office, 76–110.

Kozel, N. J. & Adams, E. H. (1986). Epidemiology of drug abuse: An overview. *Science* 234:970–974.

O'Malley, P. M., Johnston, L. D. & Bachman, J. G. (1985) Cocaine use among American adolescents and young adults. In: Kozel, N. J. & Adams, E. H. (Eds.), *Cocaine use in America: Epidemiologic and clinical perspectives*. NIDA Research Monograph 61, DHHS pub. no. (ADM) 85-1414. Washington, D.C.: Government Printing Office, 50–75.

Pasternack, P. F., Colvin, S. B. & Baumann, F. G. (1985) Cocaine-induced angina pectoris and acute myocardial infarction in patients younger than 40 years. *Am. J. Cardiol.* 55(6):847.

Raveis, V. H. & Kandel, D. B. (1987) Changes in drug behavior from the middle to the late twenties: Initiation, persistence, and cessation of use. *AJPH* 77(5):607–611.

Schachne, J. S., Roberts, B. H. & Thompson, P. D. (1984) Coronary artery spasm and myocardial infarction associated with cocaine use. *N. Engl. J. Med.* 310(25):1666.

Van Dyke, C. & Byck, R. (1982) Cocaine. *Sci. Am.* 246:128–141.

Yanagita, T. (1973) An experimental framework for evaluation of dependence liability in various types of drugs in monkeys. *Bull. Narc.* 25:57–64.

3

Neural Mechanisms of the Reinforcing Action of Cocaine

Roy A. Wise

Cocaine, like most drugs, has multiple actions. It has local anesthetic actions (Ritchie & Greene, 1985), and it amplifies the synaptic effects of the monoamines epinephrine, norepinephrine, dopamine, and serotonin in both the peripheral (Ritchie & Greene, 1985), and central (Friedman et al., 1975; Heikkila et al., 1975; Knapp & Mandell, 1972) nervous systems. The purpose of the present chapter is to summarize the evidence indicating which of these actions accounts for the habit-forming, or "reinforcing," effects of the drug.

LOCAL ANESTHETIC ACTIONS

The local anesthetic actions of cocaine appear to have little to do with its abuse liability. Several local anesthetics fail to maintain responding in animals trained to respond for cocaine reinforcement (Woolverton & Balster, 1979), and although some local anesthetics will maintain cocaine-trained responding (Ford & Balster, 1977; Johanson, 1980; Woolverton & Balster, 1979), these drugs are not known to be abused by humans (Fischman, 1984). In animal self-administration paradigms local anesthetics may sustain responding in animals trained under cocaine reinforcement, but they have not been shown to *establish* responding in untrained animals. Local anesthetics share stimulus properties with cocaine (Fischman et al., 1983) and thus the two may be confused in cocaine-trained animals. At any rate, since not all local anesthetics are self-administered by lower animals, and since noncocaine local anesthetics are not knowingly abused by humans (local anesthetics are unknowingly abused when they are sometimes used to dilute illicit cocaine), it would appear that some property of cocaine other than its local anesthetic action makes it habit forming. This conclusion is confirmed by the fact that treatments that interfere with cocaine's other actions block its reinforcing efficacy.

ACTIONS IN MONOAMINE SYSTEMS

Cocaine increases the extracellular concentration of the monoamines epinephrine, norepinephrine, dopamine, and serotonin and their metabolites. In early studies it was assumed that, like amphetamine, cocaine stimulated the release of newly synthesized monoamines (Besson et al., 1969; Farnebo & Hamberger, 1971; Knapp & Mandell, 1972; Maengwyn-Davis & Koppanyi, 1966; Moore et al., 1977; Starke & Montel, 1973; Teeters et al., 1963). However, drug-induced increases in extracellular concentration of a transmitter can result from either of two mechanisms: The drug (1) can cause release of transmitter from presynaptic nerve endings, as does amphetamine (Heikkila et al., 1975), or (2) can interfere with the inactivation of already-released transmitter by (in the case of the monoamines, at least) blocking its reuptake into the presynaptic ending (Iversen, 1967). It is now clear that cocaine is principally a reuptake blocker and not a releaser of monoamines (Heikkila et al., 1975; Ross & Reny, 1969). The physiological consequence, however, is the same: Cocaine causes higher concentrations of monoamine transmitters to reach postsynaptic monoamine receptors, thereby augmenting monoaminergic neural communication as would an agent that stimulated monoaminergic nerve firing or caused direct monoamine release from inactive presynaptic terminals.

Peripheral Autonomic Actions

Since monoamines serve as transmitters in the peripheral sympathetic nervous system, cocaine has autonomic actions (Ritchie & Greene, 1985). However, though autonomic activation accompanies cocaine self-administration, this action is not thought to contribute significantly to the abuse liability of psychomotor stimulants. First, amphetamine shares with cocaine the ability to attenuate catecholamine inactivation; in addition, amphetamine enhances synaptic release of catecholamines (Axelrod, 1970; Carlsson, 1970). Thus amphetamine, like cocaine, increases sympathetic activation by increasing the concentration of noradrenaline in peripheral synapses. However, the optical isomers of amphetamine are equally potent in the peripheral autonomic nervous system (Bromage, 1952; Northrup & Van Liere, 1953; Patil et al., 1967; Swanson et al., 1943), whereas they are differentially potent in maintaining drug self-administration (Risner, 1975; Yokel & Pickens, 1973, 1974). If peripheral sympathetic actions of amphetamine were responsible for its reinforcing effects under certain dose conditions, optical isomers should be equally effective (Davis & Smith, 1977). Finally, experimental destruction of noradrenergic systems does not alter intravenous cocaine self-administration (Roberts et al., 1977). Thus, cocaine enhances central noradrenergic function, but this enhancement does not appear to contribute to the reinforcing efficacy—and thus the abuse liability—of cocaine.

Dopaminergic Actions

The ability of cocaine to enhance the synaptic actions of dopamine is the property that seems causally linked to cocaine's abuse liability (Wise, 1984, 1987; Wise & Bozarth, 1987). Blockade of dopamine receptors with neuroleptic drugs attenuates both the reinforcing efficacy of cocaine (de Wit & Wise, 1977; Risner & Jones, 1980; Woolverton, 1986) and its rewarding efficacy (Davis & Smith, 1975; Risner & Jones, 1976; Yokel & Wise, 1975), as well as the euphoria (Gunne et al., 1972) produced by amphetamine. Direct central injections of neuroleptics into the dopamine nerve terminals of the nucleus accumbens attenuate cocaine reinforcement effectively (though not necessarily completely: Phillips, et. al., 1983). Selective neurotoxin lesions of the dopamine cells of the ventral tegmental area (Bozarth & Wise, 1986; Roberts & Koob, 1982) or of the dopamine nerve terminals of the nucleus accumbens (Lyness et al., 1979; Roberts et al., 1977, 1980) attenuate the reinforcing effects of intravenous amphetamine and cocaine in laboratory animals.

The reinforcing, or habit-forming, properties of cocaine and amphetamine can be demonstrated by direct injection of these agents into restricted regions of the brain. Two effective brain sites have been found; both are in regions of termination of dopamine pathways. Amphetamine is self-administered directly into the terminal field of the meso-accumbens dopamine pathway, thus confirming the importance of this dopamine synaptic region for amphetamine reinforcement (Hoebel et al., 1983). Cocaine injections into this region have not been found to be reinforcing (Goeders & Smith, 1983), although injections of dopamine itself have (Guerin et al., 1984). It is not clear why cocaine should not be self-administered into the nucleus accumbens, since it is believed to be an effective dopamine uptake inhibitor in this region, and since the reinforcing effects of amphetamine seem so clearly linked to this region. It is difficult to imagine how increased dopamine in the nucleus accumbens could be reinforcing when caused by amphetamine, but not when caused by cocaine. It may prove that the local anesthetic properties of cocaine are involved; perhaps cocaine blocks its own stimulant actions in the nucleus accumbens by local anesthetic actions on local output neurons.

Whatever the explanation of the failure to demonstrate reinforcing actions of cocaine in the nucleus accumbens, such actions have been demonstrated in another field of dopamine nerve terminals: the medial frontal cortex (Goeders & Smith, 1983, 1986; Goeders et al., 1986). Thus there is no doubt that cocaine is reinforcing because of actions in dopaminergic synapses, but it is not yet confirmed that the same dopaminergic synapses are involved in the reinforcing effects of amphetamine and cocaine. Amphetamine has not yet been tested to determine whether it has reinforcing effects in the frontal cortex of rats, but one such injection site in monkeys has been tested and found to support intracranial amphetamine self-administration (Phillips et al., 1981).

A test of the hypothesis that dopaminergic actions of amphetamine and cocaine give them their reinforcing actions has involved the use of selective dopamine receptor agonists. Despite the fact that these agents can also have aversive properties (Wise et al.,

1976), the dopamine agonists apomorphine, piribedil, and bromocriptine have amphetamine-like reinforcing properties in monkeys (Woolverton et al., 1984) and rats (Baxter et al., 1974, 1976; Bozarth & Wise, unpublished observations; Yokel & Wise, 1978). One of these agents, bromocriptine, alleviates cocaine craving in human addicts (Dackis & Gold, 1985a), most probably because it activates the same central mechanisms as does cocaine (reminiscent of the way that methadone satisfies, to a degree, heroin craving). Apomorphine is reinforcing even if the dopamine neurons themselves are selectively destroyed (Baxter et al., 1976), since apomorphine acts as a dopamine substitute rather than a dopamine enhancer.

Thus the abuse liability of the psychomotor stimulants is mediated through the actions of these agents on dopaminergic synaptic function. Dopamine synapses in the nucleus accumbens seem clearly involved, and dopamine synapses in the frontal cortex may also play a role. Possible roles for other dopamine synapses cannot be ruled out, and, since dopaminergic neurons pass their messages on to cells utilizing other transmitter substances, dopamine is clearly not the only neurotransmitter involved in the relevant reinforcement circuitry. Dopamine is, however, the only neurotransmitter that has thus far been identified in the circuitry of cocaine reinforcement, and it is the transmitter that identifies the anatomical sites at which cocaine *initiates* its reinforcing interaction with brain circuitry.

COMMON ACTIONS OF OPIATES

Recent evidence indicates that opiates activate the same system. Opiates are known to increase dopamine turnover (Kuschinsky & Hornykiewicz, 1972) and to accelerate the activity of mesencephalic dopamine cells (Matthews & German, 1984; Ostrowski et al., 1982). This activation is associated with the increase in locomotor activity that is caused by low doses of opiates (Babbini & Davis, 1972); increased locomotor activity can be produced by direct injections of morphine into the ventral tegmental region of dopaminergic cell bodies (Holmes & Wise, 1985; Joyce & Iversen, 1979;

Vezina & Stewart, 1984). Psychomotor activation will be mentioned later as an action common to all addictive substances.

Direct reinforcing effects of morphine can also be demonstrated when the substance is injected into the dopamine cell body region (Bozarth & Wise, 1981a 1981b; Phillips & LePiane, 1980). Animals will lever-press for such injections (Bozarth & Wise, 1981a; van Ree & de Weid, 1980),and they will return increasingly to places in the environment where such injections are experienced (Bozarth & Wise, 1981b; Phillips & LePiane, 1980). The reinforcing effects of opiates are attenuated (Bozarth & Wise, 1981b; Ettenberg et al., 1982; Spyraki et al., 1983), but not completely blocked (Ettenberg et al., 1982) by neuroleptics. Opiates can apparently activate the same brain circuitry in two places: at the level of the dopamine cell bodies of the ventral tegmental areas, and at the level of the nucleus accumbens (Goeders et al., 1984; Olds, 1982), where fibers from ventral tegmental dopamine cells terminate. Thus while most of the actions of psychomotor stimulants are distinct from those of opiates, the reinforcing actions of the two classes have common, or at least overlapping, neural mechanisms (Wise & Bozarth, 1984).

THE OPIATE DEPENDENCE MECHANISM

The common mechanism of psychomotor stimulant and opiate reinforcing actions is anatomically distinct from the neural mechanism of opiate physical dependence. Dependence is established by injections of opiates into the periaqueductal gray region (Bozarth & Wise, 1986; Wei, 1981); in animals made dependent by systemic injections of opiates, withdrawal signs can be precipitated by opiate antagonists injected into this same region. Nondependent animals do not work for morphine injections into this region (Bozarth & Wise, 1981a); dependent animals have not yet been tested. Nondependent animals will work for injections into the ventral tegmental area, however, where even continuous drug infusion fails to produce symptoms of physical dependence (Bozarth & Wise, 1986). Attempts to extend the notion of physical dependence to the psychomotor stimulants are thus unlikely to provide an explanation of

stimulant self-administration. Even opiates are powerfully rewarding for reasons unrelated to their ability to produce physical dependence.

PSYCHOMOTOR STIMULANT THEORY OF ADDICTION

If physical dependence is not a common denominator of addictive
drugs, it becomes interesting to consider other possibilities. Cocaine shares with a number of other drugs the ability to serve as a
reinforcer for lever-pressing and drug self-administration habits. Is
there a common biological mechanism for this common behavioral
property? The activation of the ventral tegmental dopamine system
emerges as a possibility, since such activation is common to reinforcing injections of cocaine and morphine—drugs that are in most
other ways quite different. The most obvious behavioral sign of
mesolimbic dopamine activation is increased locomotor activity,
and all drugs of abuse cause such activation, at least at low doses
(Wise, 1987; Wise & Bozarth, 1987). This is not surprising in drugs
that are already labeled "psychomotor" stimulants—cocaine and
amphetamine—and it is not very surprising in the case of other
stimulants like nicotine and caffeine. Each of these drugs increases
locomotor activity (Aceto & Martin, 1982; Arqueros et al., 1978;
Estler, 1979; Waldeck, 1973), and each increases dopamine turnover
(Arqueros et al., 1978; Govoni et al., 1984; Lichtensteiger et al.,
1982). It is more surprising in the case of opiates, which are generally considered depressant drugs. Opiates clearly activate locomotor
activity, however. They do so most clearly when administered centrally in the region of the dopamine cell bodies of the ventral teg-
mentum (Joyce & Iversen, 1979; Vezina & Stewart, 1984). The
sedative effects of opiates are mediated more caudally (Broekkamp
et al., 1976, 1984). Even when the drug is given systemically, so
that it reaches the mechanisms of both the stimulant and the sedative actions, psychomotor activation can be demonstrated. Although the sedative action dominates at higher doses, the
locomotor effect is seen at doses too low to cause sedation (Babbini
& Davis, 1972).

A number of other drugs of abuse share with opiates the ability to stimulate locomotor activity at low doses and the ability to sedate animals at higher doses. These drugs include ethanol (Frye & Breese, 1981), barbiturates (Jacobs & Farel, 1971), benzodiazepines (Poschel, 1971; Randall et al., 1960), and cannabis (Glick & Milloy, 1972). Phencyclidine is also a psychomotor stimulant (Castellani & Adams, 1981; Murray & Horita, 1979). Of these drugs, ethanol (Gessa et al., 1985), cannabis (Bloom, 1982), and phencyclidine (Gerhardt & Rose, 1985; Vickroy & Johnson, 1982) are known to stimulate dopamine turnover; nicotine (Arqueros et al., 1978; Giorguieff-Chesselet, 1979; Lichtensteiger et al. 1982) and caffeine (Govoni et al., 1984) stimulate dopamine turnover as well. Thus psychomotor activation—resulting from activation of mesolimbic dopamine neurons or influencing the more efferent cells with which the dopamine neurons interact—may reflect activation of a common reinforcement mechanism in the brain. Barbiturates and benzodiazepines, which activate locomotor activity without activating the dopamine system, are reasonable candidates to activate later stages of the same system.

IMPLICATIONS FOR TREATMENT

Recent attempts to develop treatment strategies for dealing with cocaine abuse have focused on cocaine craving and its possible mechanisms. Advances in our knowledge of the biological mechanisms of cocaine reinforcement and new knowledge regarding endogenous opioid receptors and opioid peptide transmitters have prompted the hope that we may soon be able to understand cocaine craving from a neurobiological perspective. Such an understanding may lead to the development of neurobiologically based treatment programs to parallel the development of methadone and clonidine treatments for opiate addiction.

That cocaine blocks dopamine reuptake suggests that chronic cocaine use may be associated with chronic dopamine depletion and consequent chronic dopamine receptor supersensitivity, and that one or both of these conditions may be associated with cocaine craving (Dackis & Gold, 1985a, 1985b; Gawin & Kleber, 1984). This hypothesis is interesting and has yet to be thoroughly tested, but it raises several questions relating to what is known about similar hypotheses as they have been advanced over the years in connection with other drugs of abuse. The notion that chronic drug use sets up an abnormal condition of excitability in the central nervous system, and that the drug is subsequently taken to relieve this condition, is an old notion, usually identified with the concept of physical dependence. That the jargon of cocaine craving is not tied to the jargon of physical dependence does not change the nature of the hypothesis. The notion that addicts take drugs to relive receptor supersensitivity has been found wanting in relation to the depressant classes for which it was originally developed (e.g., Collier, 1968; Jaffe & Sharpless, 1968). Craving for alcohol does not vary in proportion to the strength of the alcohol withdrawal syndrome; alcohol-dependent humans (Mello & Mendelson, 1972) and monkeys (Woods et al., 1971) refuse to work for alcohol during the period of most severe withdrawal stress, yet they initiate work for alcohol later, when withdrawal distress has subsided to minimal or negligible levels. Our animals will readily initiate lever-pressing for cocaine months after their last experience with the drug, when any past consequences of cocaine on dopamine levels of receptors should be expected to have long since been normalized. Indeed, we have not been able to demonstrate any dopamine depletions in our animals after near-fatal levels of chronic amphetamine or cocaine self-administration.

The most potent stimulus for drug craving appears to be a "taste" of the drug in question. Years after detoxification, ex-addicts report that a single taste of alcohol, nicotine, heroin, or cocaine prompts immediate and powerful craving for more drug. Animals that have had a history of cocaine self-administration but that have been subjected to extinction (nonreward) conditions eventually cease lever-pressing; the most powerful stimulus to reinitiate lever-pressing—despite the fact that this response is still not rewarded—is a "priming" injection or "taste" of the drug (de Wit & Stewart, 1981, 1983; Stewart, 1983; Stewart & de Wit, 1987). Whatever the contribution of dopamine depletion levels or dopamine receptor availability, signals that the drug may be available are the most salient cause of craving. The neurobiology of craving is thus likely to turn out to be more related to the neurobiology of expectation than to the neurobiology of the pharmacological aftereffects of drug use. In other words, we are far from a neurobiological understanding of cocaine craving.

The fact that we may not yet be close to a neurobiological understanding of cocaine craving does not mean that it is not a biological problem. We have clear evidence that cocaine craving develops and can be manipulated in animal species that do not have the capacity for communicating by language (Deneau et al., 1969; Stewart, 1983; Weeks, 1962). Thus cocaine craving is a biological phenomenon. However, drug craving depends very much on the past experience of the subject, and on the subject's memory for that past experience. It appears that the reinforcing actions of cocaine—and indeed, the reinforcing actions of morphine—depend more on the neuronal activity that the drug *causes* than on the neuronal activity that the drug *alleviates* (Stewart & Eikelboom, 1987). It is the subject's memory of the positive state that the drug once caused, and the hope or expectation that this state might be produced again, that would appear to explain craving for a drug that the subject knows is harmful. This seems particularly apparent in the case of nicotine, where the smoker often reports that only the first cigarette of the day really tastes good, but where nicotine craving is too strong to resist despite the desire and the medical necessity to do so. In such cases, as in cases where animals are only reinforced for a fraction of their responses, it is obvious that the memory of the last reinforcing experience is sufficient to maintain continued responding during prolonged periods of nonreinforcement. This maintained responding is presumably accompanied by, if not caused by, the craving reported by addicts who have not yet accepted the idea that they must never again experience their favorite drug.

The neurobiology of craving need not be linked to the immediate sequelae of drug withdrawal in order to be seen as a biological phenomenon. Many readers will be familiar with the unwillingness of a pet cat to go back to a diet of cat food once it has tasted canned fish. In our hope to understand the neurobiology of cocaine craving in detoxified addicts, we might well be advised to turn for a model to the fish craving of the cat who has tasted it once. In each case, it is the memory of how it "tasted" and the hope of "tasting" it again that is most likely to be the correlate of continued craving. If this view is valid, it may be that the neurobiology of craving will not be elucidated until the neurobiology of memory is better understood.

REFERENCES

Aceto, M. D. & Martin, B. R. (1982) Central actions of nicotine. *Medicinal Res. Reviews* 2:43–62.

Arqueros, L., Naquira, D. & Zunino, E. (1978) Nicotine-induced release of catecholamines from rat hippocampus and striatum. *Biochem. Pharmacol.* 27:2667–2674.

Axelrod, J. (1970) Amphetamine: Metabolism, physiological disposition, and its effects on catecholamine storage. In: Costa, E. & Garattini, S. (Eds.), *Amphetamines and related compounds.* New York: Raven Press, 207–216.

Babbini, M. & Davis, W. M. (1972) Time-dose relationships for locomotor activity effects of morphine after acute or repeated treatment. *Br. J. Pharmacol.* 46: 213–224.

Baxter, B. L., Gluckman, M. I. & Scerni, R. A. (1976) Apomorphine self-injection is not affected by alpha-methyl-paratyrosine treatment: Support for dopaminergic reward. *Physiol. Behav.* 4: 611–612.

Baxter, B. L., Gluckman, M. I., Stein, L. & Scerni, R. A. (1974) Self-injection of apomorphine in the rat: Positive reinforcement by a dopamine receptor stimulant. *Pharmacol. Biochem. Behav.* 2:387–391.

Besson, M. J., Cheramy, A., Feltz, P. & Glowinski, J. (1969) Release of newly synthesized dopamine from dopamine-containing terminals in the striatum of the rat. *Proc. Nat. Acad. Sci. USA* 62:741–748.

Bloom, A. S. (1982) Effect of Δ-9-tetrahydrocannabinol on the synthesis of dopamine and norepinephrine in mouse brain synaptosomes. *J. Pharmacol. Exp. Ther.* 221:97–103.

Bozarth, M. A. & Wise, R. A. (1981a) Heroin reward is dependent on a dopaminergic substrate. *Life Sci.* 29: 1881–1886.

Bozarth, M. A. & Wise, R. A. (1981b) Intracranial self-administration of morphine into the ventral tegmental area of rats. *Life Sci.* 28:551–555.

Bozarth, M. S. & Wise, R. A. (1986) Involvement of the ventral tegmental dopamine system in opioid and psychomotor stimulant reinforcement. In Harris, L. S. (Ed.), *Problems of drug dependence, 1985.* NIDA Research Monograph 55, DHS pub. no. (ADM) 85-1393. Washington, D.C.: Government Printing Office, 190–196.

Broekkamp, C.L.E., Van den Boggard, J. H., Heijnen, H. J., Rops, R. H., Cools, A. R. & Van Rossum, J. M. (1976) Separation of inhibiting and stimulating effects of morphine on self-stimulation behavior by intracerebral microinjections. *Eur. J. Pharmacol.* 36: 443–446.

Broekkamp, C. L., LePichon, M. & Lloyd, K. G. (1984) Akinesia after locally applied morphine near the nucleus raphé pontis of the rat. *Neurosci. Lett.* 50:313–318.

Bromage, P. R. (1952) Comparison of vasoactive drugs in man. *Br. Med. J.* 2:72–74.

Carlsson, A. (1970) Amphetamine and brain catecholamines. In: Costa, E. & Garattini, S. (Eds.), *Amphetamines and related compounds*. New York: Raven Press, 289–300.

Castellani, S. & Adams, P. M. (1981) Effects of dopaminergic drugs on phencyclidine-induced behavior in the rat. *Neuropharmacology* 20:371–374.

Collier, H.O.J. (1968) Supersensitivity and dependence. *Nature* 220: 228–231.

Dackis, C. A. & Gold, M. S. (1985a) Bromocriptine as treatment of cocaine abuse. *Lancet* 1:1151–1152.

Dackis, C. A. & Gold, M. S. (1985b) New concepts in cocaine addiction: The dopamine depletion hypothesis. *Neurosci. Biobehav. Rev.* 9:469–477.

Davis, W. M. & Smith, S. G. (1975) Effect of haloperidol on (+)-amphetamine self-administration. *J. Pharm. Pharmacol.* 27:540–542.

Davis, W. M. & Smith, S. G. (1977) Catecholaminergic mechanisms of reinforcement: Direct assessment by drug self-administration. *Life Sci.* 20:483–492.

Deneau, G., Yanagita, T. & Seevers, M. H. (1969) Self-administration of psychoactive substances by the monkey: A measure of psychological dependence. *Psychopharmacologia* 16:30–48.

de Wit, H. & Stewart, J. (1981) Reinstatement of cocaine-reinforced responding in the rat. *Psychopharmacology* 75:134–143.

de Wit, H. & Stewart, J. (1983) Drug reinstatement of heroin-reinforced responding in the rat. *Psychopharmacology* 79:29–31.

de Wit, H. & Wise, R. A. (1977) Blockade of cocaine reinforcement in rats with the dopamine receptor blocker pimozide, but not with the noradrenergic blockers phentolamine or phenoxybenzamine. *Canad. J. Psychol.* 31:195–203.

Estler, C.-J. (1979) Influence of pimozide on the locomotor activity produced by caffeine. *J. Pharm. Pharmacol.* 31:126–127.

Ettenberg, A., Pettit, H. O., Bloom, F. E. & Koob, G. F. (1982) Heroin and cocaine intravenous self-administration in rats: Mediation by separate neural systems. *Psychopharmacology* 78:204–209.

Farnebo, L-O. & Hamberger, B. (1971) Drug-induced changes in the release of H-monoamines from field stimulated rat brain slices. *Acta Physiol. cand. Suppl.* 371:35–44.

Fischman, M. W. (1984) The behavioral pharmacology of cocaine in humans. In: NIDA Research Monograph 50, DHHS pub. no. (ADM) 84-1326. Grabowski, J. (Ed.), *Cocaine: Pharmacology, effects, and treatment of abuse*. Washington, D.C.: Government Printing Office, 72–91.

Fischman, M. W., Schuster, C. R. & Hatano, Y. (1983) A comparison of the subjective and cardiovascular effects of cocaine and lidocaine in humans. *Pharmacol. Biochem. Behav.* 18:123–127.

Ford, R. D. & Balster, R. L. (1977) Reinforcing properties of intravenous procaine in rhesus monkeys. *Pharmacol. Biochem. Behav.* 6:289–296.

Friedman, E., Gershon, S. & Rotrosen, J. (1975) Effects of acute cocaine treatment on the turnover of 5-hydroxytryptamine in the rat brain. *Br. J. Pharmacol.* 54:61–64.

Frye, G. D. & Breese, G. R. (1981) An evaluation of the locomotor stimulating action of ethanol in rats and mice. *Psychopharmacology* 75:372–379.

Gawin, F. H. & Kleber, H. D. (1984) Cocaine abuse treatment: Open pilot trial with desipramine and lithium carbonate. *Arch. Gen. Psychiat.* 41:903–910.

Gerhardt, G. & Rose, G. (1985) Presynaptic action of phencyclidine (PCP) in the rat striatum defined using *in vivo* electrochemical methods. *Soc. Neurosc. Abstr.* 11:1205.

Gessa, G. L., Muntoni, F., Collu, M., Variu, L. & Mereu, G. (1985) Low doses of ethanol activate dopaminergic neurons in the ventral tegmental area. *Brain Res.* 348:201–204.

Giorguieff-Chesselet, M. F., Kemel, M. L., Wandscheer, D. & Glowinski, J. (1979) Regulation of dopamine release by presynaptic nicotinic receptors in rat striatal slices: Effect of nicotine in low concentration. *Life Sci.* 25:1257–1262.

Glick, S. D. & Milloy, S. (1972) Increased and decreased eating following THC administration. *Psychonomic Science* 29:6.

Goeders, N. E., Lane, J. D. & Smith, J. E. (1984) Self-administration of methionine enkephalin into the nucleus accumbens. *Pharmacol. Biochem. Behav.* 20:451–455.

Goeders, N. E. & Smith, J. E. (1983) Cortical dopaminergic involvement in cocaine reinforcement. *Science* 221:773–775.

Goeders, N. E. & Smith, J. E. (1986) Reinforcing properties of cocaine in the medial prefrontal cortex: Primary action on presynaptic dopaminergic terminals. *Pharmacol. Biochem. Behav.* 25:191–199.

Goeders, N. E., Sworkin, S. I. & Smith, J. E. (1986) Neuropharmacological assessment of cocaine self-administration into the medial prefrontal cortex. *Pharmacol. Biochem. Behav.* 24:1429–1440.

Govoni, S., Petkov, V. V., Montefusco, O., Missale, C., Battaini, F., Spano, P. F. & Trabucchi, M. (1984) Differential effects of caffeine on dihydroxyphenylacetic concentrations in various rat brain regions. *J. Pharm. Pharmacol.* 36:458–460.

Guerin, G. F., Goeders, N. E., Dworkin, S. I. & Smith, J. E. (1984) Intracranial self-administration of do-

pamine into the nucleus accumbens. *Soc. Neurosci. Abstr.* 10:1072.

Gunne, L. M., Anggard, E. & Jonsson, L. E. (1972) Clinical trials with amphetamine-blocking drugs. *Psychiatra Neurologia Neurochirurgia* 75:225–226.

Heikkila, R. E., Orlansky, H. & Cohen, G. (1975) Studies on the distinction between uptake inhibition and release of (^{3}H)dopamine in rat brain tissue slices. *Biochem. Pharmacol.* 24:847–852.

Hoebel, B. G., Monaco, A., Hernandes, L., Aulisi, E., Stanley, B. G. & Lenard, L. (1983) Self-injection of amphetamine directly into the brain. *Psychopharmacology* 81:158–163.

Holmes, L. J. & Wise, R. A. (1985) Contralateral circling induced by tegmental morphine: Anatomical localization, pharmacological specificity, and phenomenology. *Brain Res.* 326:19–26.

Iversen, L. L. (1967) *The uptake and storage of noradrenaline in sympathetic nerves.* London: Cambridge University Press.

Jacobs, B. L. & Farel, P. B. (1971) Motivated behavior produced by incresed arousal in the presence of goal objects. *Physiol. Behav.* 6:473–476.

Jaffe, J. H. & Sharpless, S. K. (1968) Pharmacological denervation supersensitivity in the central nervous system: A theory of physical dependence. In: Wikler, A. H., (Ed.), *The addictive states.* Baltimore: Williams and Wilkins, 226–246.

Johanson, C. E. (1980) The reinforcing properties of procaine, chloroprocaine and proparacaine in rhesus monkeys. *Psychopharmacology* 67:189–194.

Joyce, E. M. & Iversen, S. D. (1979) The effect of morphine applied locally to mesencephalic dopamine cell bodies on spontaneous motor activity in the rat. *Neurosci. Lett.* 14:207–212.

Knapp, S. & Mandell, A. J. (1972)

Narcotic drugs: Effects on the serotonin biosynthetic systems of the brain. *Science* 177:1209–1211.

Kuschinsky, K. & Hornykiewicz, O. (1972) Morphine catalepsy in the rat: Relation to striatal dopamine metabolism. *Eur. J. Pharmacol.* 19:119–122.

Lichtensteiger, W., Hefti, F., Felix, D., Huwyler, T., Melamed, E. & Schlumpf, M. (1982) Stimulation of nigrostriatal dopamine neurones by nicotine. *Neuropharmacology* 21:963–968.

Lyness, W. H., Friedle, N. M. & Moore, K. E. (1979) Destruction of dopaminergic nerve terminals in nucleus accumbens: Effect on d-amphetamine self-administration. *Pharmacol. Biochem. Behav.* 11:553–556.

Maengwyn-Davis, G. D. & Koppanyi, T. (1966) Cocaine tachyphylaxis and effects on indirectly acting sympathomimetic drugs in the rabbit aortic strip and in splenic tissue. *J. Pharmacol. Exp. Ther.* 154:481–492.

Matthews, R. T. & German, D. C. (1984) Electrophysiological evidence for excitation of rat ventral tegmental area dopaminergic neurons by morphine. *Neuroscience* 11:617–626.

Mello, N. K. & Mendelson, J. H. (1972) Drinking patterns during work-contingent and non-contingent alcohol acquisition. *Psychosom. Med.* 34:139–164.

Moore, K. E., Chiueh, C. C. & Zeldes, G. (1977) Release of neurotransmitters from the brain *in vivo* by amphetamine, methylphenidate and cocaine. In: Ellinwood, E. H. & Kilbey, M. M., (Eds.), *Cocaine and other stimulants.* New York: Plenum Press, 143–160.

Murray, T. F. & Horita, A. (1979) Phencyclidine-induced stereotyped behavior in rats: Dose response effects and antagonism by neuroleptics. *Life Sci.* 24: 2217–2226.

Olds, M. E. (1982) Reinforcing effects of morphine in the nucleus accumbens. *Brain Res.* 237:429–440.

Ostrowski, N. L., Hatfield, C. B. & Caggiula, A. R. (1982) The effects of low doses of morphine on the activity of dopamine containing cells and on behavior. *Life Sci.* 31:2347–2350.

Northrup, D. W. & Van Liere, E. J. (1953) Effect of the isomers of amphetamine and desoxyephedrine on gastric empying in man. *J. Pharmacol. Exp. Ther.* 109:358–360.

Patil, P. N., LaPidus, J. B., Campbell, D. & Tye, A. (1967) Steric aspects of adrenergic drugs. II. Effects of *dl* isomers and desoxy derivatives on the reserpine-pretreated vas deferens. *J. Pharmacol. Exp. Ther.* 155:13–23.

Phillips, A. G., Broekkamp, C.L.E. & Fibiger, H. C. (1983) Strategies for studying the neurochemical substrates of drug reinforcement in rodents. *Prog. Neuro-Psychopoharmacol. Biol. Psychiat.* 7:585–590.

Phillips, A. G. & LePiane, F. G. (1980) Reinforcing effects of morphine microinjection into the ventral tegmental area. *Pharmacol. Biochem. Behav.* 12: 965–968.

Phillips, A. G., Mora, F. & Rolls, E. T. (1981) Intracerebral self-administration of amphetamine by rhesus monkeys. *Neurosci. Lett.* 24:81–86.

Poschel, B.P.H. (1971) A simple and specific screen for benzodiazepine-like drugs. *Psychopharmacologia* 19:193–198.

Randall, L. O., Schallek, W., Heise, G. A., Keith, E. F. & Bagdon, R. E. (1960) The psychosedative properties of methaminodiazepoxide. *J. Pharmacol. Exp. Ther.* 129:163–171.

Risner, M. E. (1975) Intravenous self-administration of d- and 1-amphetamine by dog. *Eur. J. Pharmacol.* 32: 344–348.

Risner, M. E. & Jones, B. E. (1976) Role of noradrenergic and dopaminergic processes in amphetamine self-administration. *Pharmacol. Biochem. Behav.* 5:477–482.

Risner, M. E. & Jones, B. E. (1980) Intravenous self-administration of cocaine and norcocaine by dogs. *Psychopharmacology* 71:83–89.

Ritchie, J. M. & Greene, N. M. (1985) Local anesthetics. In: Gilman, A. G., Goodman, L. S., Rall, T. W., & Murad, F. (Eds.), *The pharmacological basis of therapeutics,* New York: Macmillan, 302–321.

Roberts, D.C.S., Corcoran, M. E. & Fibiger, H. C. (1977) On the role of ascending catecholaminergic systems in intravenous self-administration of cocaine. *Pharmacol. Biochem. Behav.* 6: 615–620.

Roberts, D.C.S. & Koob, G. (1982) Disruption of cocaine self-administration following 6-hydroxydopamine lesions of the ventral tegmental area in rats. *Pharmacol. Biochem. Behav.* 17:901–904.

Roberts, D.C.S., Koob, G. F., Klonoff, P. & Fibiger, H. C. (1980) Extinction and recovery of cocaine self-administration following 6-OHDA lesions of the nucleus accumbens. *Pharmacol. Biochem. Behav.* 12:781–787.

Ross, S. B. & Renyi, A. L. (1969) Inhibition of the uptake of tritiated 5-hydroxytryptamine in brain tissue. *Eur. J. Pharmacol.* 7:270–277.

Spyraki, C., Fibiger, H. C. & Phillips, A. G. (1983) Attenuation of heroin reward in rats by disruption of the mesolimbic dopamine system. *Psychopharmacology* 79:278–283.

Starke, K. & Montel, H. (1973) Alpha-receptor-mediated modulation of transmitter release from central noradrenergic neurones. *Naunyn-Schmiedeberg's Arch. Pharmacol.* 279:53–60.

Stewart, J. (1983) Conditioned and unconditioned drug effects in relapse to opiate and stimulant drug self-administration. *Prog. Neuro-Psychopharmacol. Biol. Psychiat.* 7:591–597.

Stewart, J. & de Wit, H. (1987) Reinstatement of drug-taking behavior as a method of assessing incentive motivational properties of drugs. In: Bozarth, M. A. (Ed.), *Methods of assessing the reinforcing properties of abused drugs.* New York: Springer-Verlag.

Stewart, J. & Eikelboom, R. (1987) Conditioned drug effects. In: Iversen, L. L., Iversen, S. D., & Snyder, S. H., (Eds.), *Handbook of psychopharmacology,* vol. 19, 1–57.

Swanson, E. E., Scott, C. C., Lee, H. M. & Chen, K. K. (1943) Comparison of the pressor action of some optical isomers of sympathomimetic amines. *J. Pharmacol. Exp. Ther.* 79:329–333.

Teeters, W. R., Koppanyi, T. & Cowan, F. F. (1963) Cocaine tachyphylaxis. *Life Sci.* 2:509–518.

van Ree, J. M. & de Wied, D. (1980) Involvement of neurohypophyseal peptides in drug-mediated adaptive responses. *Pharmacol. Biochem. Behav.* 13 (Suppl. 1):257–263.

Vezina, P. & Stewart, J. (1984) Conditioning and place-specific sensitization of increases in activity induced by morphine in the VTA. *Pharmacol. Biochem. Behav.* 20:925–929.

Vickroy, T. W. & Johnson, K. M. (1982) Similar dopamine-releasing effects of phencyclidine and nonamphetamine stimulants in striatal slices. *J. Pharmacol. Exp. Ther.* 223:669–674.

Waldeck, B. (1973) Modification of caffeine-induced locomotor stimulation by a cholinergic mechanism. *J. Neural Trans.* 34:61–72.

Weeks, J. R. (1962) Experimental morphine addiction: Method for automatic intravenous injections in unrestrained rats. *Science* 138:143–144.

Wei, E. (1981) Enkephaline analogs and physical dependence. *J. Pharmacol. Exp. Ther.* 216:12–18.

Wise, R. A. (1984) Neural mechanisms of the reinforcing action of cocaine. In: Grabowski, J. (Ed.), *Cocaine: Pharmacology, effects, and treatment of abuse.* NIDA Research Monograph 50, DHHS pub. no. (ADM) 84-1326. Washington, D.C.: Government Printing Office, 15–33.

Wise, R. A. (1987) The role of reward pathways in the development of drug dependence. *Pharmacol. Ther.* 35:227–263.

Wise, R. A. & Bozarth, M. A. (1984) Brain reward circuitry: Four circuit elements "wired" in apparent series. *Brain Res. Bull.* 297:265–273.

Wise, R. A. & Bozarth, M. A. (1987) A psychomotor stimulant theory of addiction. *Psychol. Rev.* 94:469–492.

Wise, R. A., Yokel, R. A. & de Wit, H. (1976) Both positive reinforcement and conditioned taste aversion from amphetamine and from apomorphine in rats. *Science* 191:1273–1274.

Woods, J. H., Ikomi, F. & Winger, G. (1971) The reinforcing properties of ethanol. In: Roach, M. K., McIsaac, W. M., & Creaven, P. J. (Eds.), *Biological aspects of alcoholism.* Austin: University of Texas Press, 371–388.

Woolverton, W. L. (1986) Effects of a D_1 and a D_2 Dopamine antagonist on the self-administration of cocaine and piribedil by rhesus monkeys. *Pharmacol. Biochem. Behav.* 24:531–535.

Woolverton, W. L. & Balster, R. L. (1979) Reinforcing properties of some local anesthetics in rhesus monkeys. *Pharmacol. Biochem. Behav.* 11:669–672.

Woolverton, W. L., Goldberg, L. I. & Ginos, J. (1984) Intravenous self-administration of dopamine receptor agonists by rhesus monkeys. *J. Pharmacol. Exp. Ther.* 230:678–683.

Yokel, R. A. & Pickens, R. (1973) Self-administration of optical isomers of amphetamine and methylamphetamine by rats. *J. Pharmacol. Exp. Ther.* 187:27–33.

Yokel, R. A. & Pickens, R. (1974) Drug level of *d*- and *l*- amphetamine during intravenous self-administration. *Psychopharmacologia* 34:255–264.

Yokel, R. A. & Wise, R. A. (1975) Increased lever pressing for amphetamine after pimozide in rats: Implications for a dopamine theory of reward. *Science* 187:547–549.

Yokel, R. A. & Wise, R. A. (1976) Attenuation of intravenous amphetamine reinforcement by central dopamine blockade in rats. *Psychopharmacology* 48:311–318.

Yokel, R. A. & Wise, R. A. (1978) Amphetamine-type reinforcement by dopamine agonists in the rat. *Psychopharmacology* 58:289–296.

4

Cocaine: Synaptic Effects and Adaptations

Alan C. Swann

INTERPRETATION OF BASIC NEURAL EFFECTS OF COCAINE

The profound behavioral effects of cocaine are eventually related to its actions at the synapse. As described by Wise in this volume, among the behavioral effects is activation of an elegant reward system that normally ensures behavior necessary for survival of the individual or species. The adaptations that occur in these neural systems have clear biological importance. Cocaine stimulates the reward system so powerfully that it can supplant other rewards that are vital. It is important to understand why cocaine, which appears only moderately effective in its individual synaptic actions, is such an effective drug, and why the sensitivity to many of its actions increases progressively with repeated exposure to the drug.

This chapter will examine the synaptic effects of cocaine and the adaptations to them that might occur. Behavioral effects of cocaine have generally been interpreted in terms of single transmitter effects, and there is little information about the role of transmitter interactions. In addition, though the local anesthetic effect of cocaine appears not to be a primary cause of its behavioral effects, it will almost certainly modify the transmitter adaptations to repeated treatment.

Examination of the information now available about relationships between behavioral and neural effects of cocaine raises several questions:

1. What is the correlation between the behavior effects of cocaine and its inhibition of dopamine, norepinephrine, and serotonin reuptake, and how does cocaine compare with other drugs that overlap in terms of transmitter effects?

2. What adaptive changes take place in neurotransmitter availability during repeated cocaine treatment?

3. What role do local anesthetic effects of cocaine have in its behavioral effects and in the adaptation to repeated treatment?

4. What is the influence of interactions among direct effects of cocaine on norepinephrine, dopamine, and serotonin on the acute and chronic effects of the drug?

5. What are the roles of indirect effects on transmitters such as acetylcholine and gamma-aminobutyric acid (GABA), and on peptide and neuroendocrine systems?

6. What neurophysiologic changes occur during repeated exposure to cocaine, and what is their role in the progressive sensitization to some of its effects, and their relationship to kindling phenomena?

This chapter will focus on current information about these questions. After a brief overview of relationships between synaptic and behavioral effects of cocaine, we will discuss direct synaptic effects in vitro, acute effects on neurotransmitter economy and neural activity, adaptations to repeated exposure to cocaine, neurophysiologic effects and their relationship to kindling, and primary and secondary transmitter interactions during cocaine treatment.

SYNAPTIC EFFECTS OF COCAINE AND BEHAVIOR

Although cocaine has been known as a stimulant for centuries, the local anesthetic properties of cocaine were responsible for its original interest to Western medicine (Cregler & Mark, 1986; Freud, 1884; Holmstedt & Fregda, 1981). Similar to other local anesthetics, cocaine inhibits transport through the voltage-sensitive Na^+ channel (Ritchie & Greene, 1985). The EC_{50} for this effect is about 1–10 μM, similar to that for inhibition of monoamine reuptake (Mathews & Collins, 1983). The activity profile for local anesthetic effects among cocaine congeners does not resemble that for most behavioral effects of cocaine (Mathews & Collins, 1983).

Behavioral Effects of Cocaine and Dopaminergic Systems

Behavioral effects of cocaine have generally been interpreted in terms of the role of dopamine. Self-administration of cocaine is prevented by lesions with the catecholamine neurotoxin 6-hydroxydopamine (Roberts et al., 1977), and cocaine-induced stereotypy and hyperkinesis are prevented by monoamine depletion with reserpine (Sayers & Handley, 1973) or by 6-hydroxydopamine lesions of dopaminergic tracts (Creese & Iverson, 1975; Pettit et al., 1984). Blockade of postsynaptic D2 dopamine receptors also reduces cocaine self-administration (Goeders & Smith, 1986).

There are several discrete systems of dopaminergic neurons in the brain (Moore & Bloom, 1978). The nigrostriatal system projects from cell bodies in the substantia nigra to the corpus striatum. The mesolimbic and mesocortical systems project from cell bodies in the ventral tegmental area to the nucleus accumbens, olfactory tubercle, and other limbic forebrain regions or to the prefrontal cortex, respectively. Smaller systems with primarily endocrine functions include the tuberoinfundibular and tuberohypophyseal systems, which project to the median eminence and posterior pituitary, the incertohypothalamic system, and the paraventricular system. Although dopaminergic regulation varies among these systems, as will be discussed in a later section, sensitivity of reuptake to cocaine in vitro is similar (Hadfield & Nugent, 1983).

Increased transmission in the mesolimbic and mesocortical systems, which include the ventral tegmental area, median forebrain bundle, nucleus accumbens, and other limbic forebrain regions, is consistent with the well-documented enhancement of reward mechanisms by cocaine (Dworkin & Smith, 1986; Goeders & Smith, 1983; Wise, 1980). Animals will self-administer cocaine directly into the prefrontal cortex, but not into other dopaminergic brain regions (Goeders & Smith, 1983, 1986). The role of different mesocortical brain areas may differ between the initiation and maintenance of cocaine self-administration. Although the medial prefrontal cortex is clearly important in acute cocaine self-administration, Martin-Iversen et al. (1986) found that destruction of dopaminergic terminals in the medial prefrontal had no effect on cocaine self-administration that was already established. Destruction of postsynaptic neurons in the nucleus accumbens, however, reduced established cocaine self-administration (Zito et al., 1985).

The mesocortical effects seem most prominent in terms of self-administration (Goeders & Smith, 1983, 1986; Morency et al., 1987) and place conditioning (Morency & Beninger, 1986). This is of interest in the context of dopaminergic regulation because autoreceptors are relatively sparse in the mesocortical compared to the mesolimbic and nigrostriatal systems (Bannon & Roth, 1983), dopaminergic innervation of the medial prefrontal area is sparse relative to noradrenergic and serotonergic inputs (Lane et al., 1982; Moore & Bloom, 1978), and the mesocortical system may be especially sensitive to stress (Thierry et al., 1976)

The nigrostriatal system is involved in dopamine effects on extrapyramidal systems; increased transmission results in hyperkinesia and stereotypy and can lead to dyskinetic or choreoform movement disorders. Cocaine administration is associated with hyperkinesia and stereotypy in rats (Pradhan et al., 1978), and these effects appear to be localized to the corpus striatum (Swerdlow et al, 1986).

The tuberoinfundibular system is involved in endocrine modulation, particularly inhibition of prolactin release (McLeod & Login, 1976). This, however, has not been associated with cocaine use; in fact, cocaine increases prolactin (Dackis et al., 1984). Increased prolactin release by other stimulants (Halbreich et al., 1981) has been attributed to increased serotonin release (Halbreich et al., 1981; Kuhn et al., 1981). As discussed later, cocaine appears to inhibit serotonergic transmission (Pradhan et al., 1978), so the explanation for the prolactin effect is not clear.

An additional neuroendocrine action of dopamine is the regulation of TSH (thyroid-stimulating hormone) release (Jackson, 1982). The TSH response to TRH (thyrotropin-releasing hormone) is blunted in chronic cocaine users (Giannini et al, 1987), consistent with increased dopaminergic activity (Loosen & Prange, 1982).

Behavioral effects of cocaine are therefore consistent with functionally increased dopamine. Neuroendocrine effects are mixed, suggesting that net effects on dopaminergic transmission differ among dopaminergic systems or that other transmitter effects are also involved.

Role of Norepinephrine and Serotonin in Behavior Effects

If cocaine inhibits norepinephrine and serotonin reuptake, then cocaine use would be expected to lead to functional increases in these transmitters. Increased noradrenergic transmission is associated with increased arousal, which has been observed with cocaine use (Scheel-Kruger et al., 1977); noradrenergic transmission is also increased in mania and correlates with euphoria (dopamine does not) (Swann et al., 1987). Cocaine-induced euphoria may similarly have a noradrenergic substrate (Gawin, 1986). The antagonistic effects of cocaine and alcohol on anxiety presumably involve norepinephrine (Aston-Jones et al., 1984). Increased noradrenergic function therefore may also have a role in the acute effects of cocaine.

The expected results of increased serotonergic transmission include increased sleep, inhibition of aggression, and complex endocrine effects. The effects of cocaine are generally the opposite. Cocaine, in fact, reduces the turnover and rate of synthesis of serotonin, with consistent behavioral effects (Friedman et al., 1975; Pradhan et al., 1978; Schubert et al., 1979). This inhibitory effect on serotonergic transmission may be due to reduced synthesis (Knapp & Mandell, 1972) combined with receptor antagonism (Fozard et al., 1979).

Behavioral and neuroendocrine effects of acute cocaine are therefore consistent with increased noradrenergic transmission, increased dopaminergic transmission at least in most of its systems, and decreased serotonergic transmission despite the similar reuptake effects on these three transmitters. Examination of the effects of cocaine in vitro in more detail may yield information about reasons for these differences, about the nature of the adaptations to repeated exposure to cocaine, and about possible differences between cocaine and other stimulants.

EFFECTS OF COCAINE IN VITRO

Approaches to Measuring Effects of Cocaine and Their Relevance to Brain Function

A host of measures for effects on all phases of synaptic function in vitro is available. Membrane effects can be measured by effects on membrane fluidity at depths associated with different membrane components (Chapman & Hayward, 1985) and by effects on movements of ions through channels with specific antagonists. Effects on transmitter function can be measured by effects on enzymes of transmitter synthesis, transmitter storage, release, reuptake, inactivation, receptor binding, and second messenger effects consequent to receptor binding including adenylate or guanylate cyclase and phosphoinositide turnover. Interactions between cocaine and some of these systems have been examined. Primary effects on one of these systems will, of course, be likely to produce secondary effects on others.

Effects on the Cell Membrane

Cocaine inhibits impulse propagation by blocking Na^+ influx through its voltage-sensitive channel (Mathews & Collins, 1983). The anesthetic effect of cocaine is not considered responsible for its effects on reward, because they are not shared by other drugs with similar membrane effects (Woolverton & Balster, 1979). However, though animals will not generally learn to self-administer local anesthetics, learned self-administration of cocaine can generalize to local anesthetics (see the chapter by Wise). In addition, local anesthetic effects contribute to other neurophysiologic effects of cocaine and modify some of its transmitter effects (discussed in a later section).

Effects on Synaptic Function

The synaptic actions of cocaine include (1) direct effects in vitro on the basic phases of transmitter synthesis, storage, release, and inactivation; (2) secondary effects that become evident when cocaine is given acutely in vivo; and (3) adaptations to repeated cocaine administration, including those of interactions among the affected transmitters. These effects will be examined in the following sections.

Release and Reuptake of Neurotransmitters

Cocaine inhibits the reuptake of norepinephrine, dopamine, and serotonin (Banerjee et al., 1987; Hadfield & Nugent, 1983; Hoffman et al., 1986; Ross & Renyi, 1967). This, in turn, blocks the major pathway of their inactivation and would be expected to increase their availability at the synapse. The effect is competitive with transmitter, with K_i for cocaine of about 1 μM (Banerjee et al., 1987). The potency of the effect is similar for the three transmitters, perhaps somewhat stronger for serotonin (Ross & Renyi, 1969). Although the IC_{50} for inhibition of dopamine uptake by cocaine is similar in the corpus striatum (nigrostriatal system), olfactory tubercle (mesolimbic system), and prefrontal cortex (mesocortical system), both the prefrontal cortex and olfactory tubercle have about 25% cocaine-insensitive dopamine reuptake, whereas the striatum does not (Hadfield & Nugent, 1983).

The results of inhibition of norepinephrine uptake by cocaine have been compared to those of desipramine in several systems. In the hippocampus, low concentrations of cocaine potentiate effects of added norepinephrine, similar to desipramine; higher concentrations have a depressant effect similar to local anesthetics (Yasuda et al., 1984). Cocaine has a similar biphasic effect on stimulation-induced norepinephrine release in the atrium, which is increased by desipramine (Lew & Angus, 1983). Cocaine and desipramine have opposite effects on stimulation-induced norepinephrine overflow in the heart (Dart et al., 1983). Effects of cocaine on synaptic norepinephrine are therefore not comparable to pure reuptake blockers due to cocaine's local anesthetic effects. In addition, cocaine may interact directly with alpha-2 receptors (Pelayo et al., 1980).

Neurotransmitter Storage and Metabolism

Due to its inhibition of transmitter reuptake, cocaine reduces presynaptic concentrations of transmitter. Cocaine does not appear to affect monoamine oxidase directly, but its secondary effects are complex and will be described in the section on effects of cocaine in vivo.

Neurotransmitter Synthesis

The rate-limiting enzymes for norepinephrine, dopamine, and serotonin synthesis are regulated in part by product inhibition, leading to a potential increase in activity during cocaine treatment due to reduced reuptake of transmitter. In addition, however, the synthesis of these amines requires uptake of precursor amino acid into the cell. Serotonin is particularly sensitive to this effect; serotonin synthesis under most conditions may actually be limited by the supply of tryptophan (Milner & Wurtman, 1986; Swann et al., 1981). Cocaine has been reported to inhibit high-affinity tryptophan uptake (Knapp & Mandell, 1972), which may contribute to its overall inhibitory effects on serotonergic function.

In contrast to its effects on serotonin, cocaine may increase dopamine synthesis in addition to inhibiting its reuptake. Bagchie and Reilly (1983) reported that cocaine increased the synthesis of dopamine from radiolabeled phenylalanine or tyrosine (Bagchie, 1985) in crude synaptosomes from rat caudate, without affecting the uptake of labeled precursor. This was inhibited by reserpine, similar to the case with the stimulants amfonelic acid (Bagchie et al., 1980) and methylphenidate (Bagchie, 1985). By contrast, d-amphetamine increased the release of newly synthesized dopamine but did not increase dopamine synthesis from precursors. Cocaine may therefore stimulate tyrosine hydroxylase by disrupting the relationship between dopamine synthesis and storage (Bagchie, 1985).

There is no information about whether cocaine can stimulate norepinephrine synthesis similarly in synaptosomes from regions with major noradrenergic innervation. If the stimulation results from interference with the vesicular storage of transmitter as suggested by Bagchie (1985), the effect on norepinephrine might be similar since its uptake into storage vesicles appears identical (Slotkin et al., 1978).

Cocaine Binding Sites

Properties of synaptic binding sites for cocaine may provide information about the mechanism, specificity, or adaptive changes in its effects. Cocaine binding has been described in membranes from several brain regions (Reith et al., 1984). Sodium-dependent binding in the corpus striatum is reduced in Parkinson's disease (Pimoule et al., 1983) and appears to be associated with dopamine reuptake sites (Kennedy & Hanbauer, 1983). Other stimulants competitively inhibit cocaine binding; binding correlates roughly with dopamine concentrations across brain regions; and binding is reduced by 6-hydroxydopamine under conditions where it destroys presynaptic dopaminergic terminals, but not by the postsynaptic neurotoxin kainic acid (Kennedy & Hanbauer, 1983; Sershen et al. 1980). Sershen et al. (1984) reported that the dopaminergic toxin MTPP reduced sodium-dependent binding and dopamine uptake in the corpus striatum, but did not alter Na^+-dependent cocaine binding in the olfactory tubercle. The significance of sodium-dependent cocaine binding outside the nigrostriatal system is therefore not clear.

Sodium-independent binding in the cerebral cortex appears related to serotonin uptake sites, since it is reduced by serotonin depletion with p-chlorophenylalanine or with 5,7-dihydroxytryptamine (Reith et al., 1983, 1984). The binding sites for cocaine and imipramine are not identical, since they differ in sensitivity to inhibitors, number of sites (about fivefold more cocaine binding sites), and mechanism of inhibition by the other drug (Reith et al., 1984). There is no information about adaptive changes in these binding sites during administration of cocaine or other drugs, or about the relationship to norepinephrine reuptake sites. Ritz et al. (1987) reported that the ability of drugs to bind to the cocaine binding site inhibiting dopamine uptake correlated with self-administration.

Significance of Neural Activity and Possible Adaptive Mechanisms

Effects on uptake of neurotransmitters or their precursors do not occur in a vacuum. If synaptic transmitter concentrations are increased by reuptake blockade, adaptations in the presynaptic cell could include the following:

1. Decreased firing rate and synthesis due to increased auto-receptor binding (El Mestikawy et al., 1986; Fuder et al., 1984; Hoffmann & Cubeddu, 1984; McMillen, 1982; Pitts & Marwah, 1987)

2. Increased synthesis due to decreased intrasynaptic transmitter concentration, since the rate-limiting enzymes are regulated in part by product inhibition (Demarest & Moore, 1979), and due possibly to phosphorylation of tyrosine hydroxylase (Lazar et al., 1982)

3. Decreased activity of degradative enzymes due to reduced concentration of transmitter.

The long-term effect would depend on the balance between the above effects and the availability of precursor (Milner & Wurtman, 1985) and on anatomic location: Autoreceptors may be relatively scarce or absent in the mesocortical (Bannon et al., 1981) and tuber-oinfundibular (Demarest & Moore, 1979) compared to the meso-limbic and nigrostriatal systems, and cholinergic and GABAergic feedback loops are better developed in the nigrostriatal than in the other systems (Clark et al., 1985a, 1985b). These differences may be particularly relevant to cocaine effects given the importance of the mesocortical system in cocaine self-administration (Goeders & Smith, 1983, 1986).

Adaptations in the postsynaptic cell would depend, in turn, on the overall effect on integrated synaptic activity. If transmitter were depleted, for example, the postsynaptic response would include in-creased receptor number and, perhaps, sensitivity.

Any of these adaptations could be altered by the inhibition by cocaine of voltage-dependent Na^+ influx. The effect of dopamine autoreceptors also appears to involve this mechanism (Hoffmann & Cubeddu, 1984), and presumably could therefore be reduced by co-caine.

APPROACHES TO COCAINE EFFECTS IN VIVO

Although interpretation is more complex than in the case of experi-mentation in vitro, a more integrated view of the effects of cocaine can be obtained after the drug is given acutely or chronically to intact animals. Data obtained in vitro, however, are then helpful in distinguishing primary from secondary effects.

Effects of Acute Treatment on Monoamine Neurotransmitters

Acute treatment with cocaine, at doses with behavioral effects, initially increases the synaptic concentrations of dopamine and norepinephrine (Pradhan, 1983; Pradhan et al., 1978). This reduces the firing rate of noradrenergic cells in the locus coeruleus after relatively small doses of cocaine, due to increased binding of norepinephrine to autoreceptors (Pitts & Marwah, 1986). Binding of dopamine to norepinephrine autoreceptors probably contributes to this effect (Jackisch et al., 1985; Misu et al., 1985). Indices of serotonin release and turnover, however, are reduced from the start (Pradhan et al., 1978), in contrast to the increased serotonin turnover after a single dose of amphetamine or iprindole (Warren et al., 1984).

Treatment with cocaine alters enzymes of monoamine synthesis and degradation in a manner generally consistent with the above effects. Acute cocaine increases activity of tyrosine hydroxylase, the rate-limiting enzyme in dopamine and norepinephrine synthesis, followed in 20 minutes by decreased activity (Pradhan, 1983). Tryptophan hydroxylase, which is rate-limiting for serotonin synthesis, is decreased after acute cocaine (Pradhan, 1983). Acute cocaine decreases monoamine oxidase activity within 10 minutes with increased activity at 20 minutes and return to normal at 40 minutes. This effect is most prominent for type A, the more important form in degradation of norepinephrine, dopamine, and serotonin (Pradhan, 1983). These time-dependent effects on enzymes of monoamine synthesis and degradation may make effects of cocaine on concentrations of individual amines or metabolites difficult to interpret. The increase in synaptically produced 3-methoxytyramine (DiGiulio et al., 1978) combined with decreased intraneuronally produced homovanillic acid (Fekete & Borsy, 1971) after administration of acute cocaine is consistent, however, with blockade of reuptake into presynaptic terminals. Demonstration of these effects generally requires doses of 10–30 mg/kg (Pradhan, 1983).

Despite the similarity across brain regions in the inhibition of dopamine reuptake by cocaine, administration in vivo has variable effects. A single injection of cocaine (20 mg/kg) has been reported to inhibit dopamine reuptake in the corpus striatum, whereas either acute or repeated treatment (21 days) increased dopamine reuptake in the nucleus accumbens (Missale et al, 1985). This may account for variations in receptor changes during chronic cocaine (discussed in a later section).

Effects of Acute Treatment on Neural Activity

There is, perhaps surprisingly, relatively little information about the effects of cocaine on the firing of spontaneously active neurons. Acute intravenous treatment with cocaine decreases the firing rate of identified noradrenergic cells in the locus coeruleus (Pitts & Marwah, 1986), serotonergic cells in the dorsal raphe (Cunningham & Lakoski, 1988), and dopaminergic cells in the ventral tegmental area and zona compacta of the substantia nigra, without altering characteristics of the action potentials (Pitts & Marwah, 1987). Cocaine activated postsynaptic noradrenergic cerebellar Purkinje neurons, and did not potentiate their inhibition by locus coeruleus stimulation. Effects of cocaine on presynaptic neurons were antagonized by autoreceptor blockers or reserpine. Procaine did not share these effects. The effects on presynaptic cells were therefore consistent with transmitter reuptake blockade, but those on postsynaptic cells appeared more complex (Pitts & Marwah, 1987).

Adaptations to Repeated Treatment in Dopaminergic Systems

When cocaine is given repeatedly, the following types of adaptations can occur: (1) homeostatic changes within each of the affected transmitter systems, including responses to stimulation combined with eventual depletion if the rate of transmitter synthesis is inadequate; (2) long-term effects of Na^+ channel blockade; (3) interactions among the transmitters directly affected by cocaine; and (4) secondary effects on other transmitter systems. We will first consider the factors influencing adaptation within dopaminergic systems.

Synthetic Pools of Dopamine and their Sensitivity to Depletion of Substrate.

Unlike norepinephrine, dopamine appears to have two storage pools: One consists of recently synthesized transmitter and is relatively sensitive to alpha-methylparatyrosine; the other, a vesicular storage pool, turns over more slowly and is depleted by reserpine (Lawson-Wendling et al., 1981). Repeated treatment with cocaine appears to deplete the reserpine-sensitive pool, since cocaine-induced behavioral and neurophysiologic effects are prevented by reserpine but not by alpha-methyltyrosine (Davis, 1985; Scheel-Kruger et al., 1977). This is similar to the case with amfonelic acid and methylphenidate, but opposite to d-amphetamine (Lawson-Wendling et al., 1981).

Role of Autoreceptors and their Relationship to Distribution.

Presynaptic dopaminergic autoreceptors exert negative feedback control on dopamine synthesis and release. They would be expected to have an important role in any long-term changes in dopaminergic activity. Autoreceptors are unequally distributed among dopaminergic systems, however, and are reported to be relatively sparse or absent in the tuberoinfundibular (Demarest & Moore, 1979) and mesocortical systems (Bannon et al., 1981). The latter may explain the relatively weak effect of cocaine on the firing of dopaminergic neurons that innervate the nucleus accumbens (Einhorn et al., 1988).

Receptor Adaptations.

Consistent with the depletion of dopamine, repeated cocaine treatment (10 or 20 mg/kg/day for 7 or 14 days) increased the number of spiperone binding sites (preynaptic and postsynaptic D2 receptors) in the corpus striatum (Taylor et al., 1979). This resulted in increased sensitivity to episodic bursts of dopamine release (Dackis & Gold, 1985). More recently, however, 15 days of treatment with 10 mg/kg/day cocaine was reported to increase postsynaptic D2 receptor number (sulpiride binding) in the nucleus accumbens but to decrease it in the corpus striatum; the investigators verified these results with quantitative autoradiography (Goeders & Kuhar, 1987). These results were consistent with the effects on dopamine reuptake described above (Missale et al., 1985), and emphasize the importance of possible regional variations in dopaminergic regulation (Clark et al., 1985b; Demarest & Moore, 1979; Kornhuber & Kornhuber, 1986). Experimental conditions are also important: In the experiments of Taylor et al. (1979), rats were killed two days after the last cocaine dose, so effects of cocaine withdrawal may have been involved. The tissue used by Goeders and Kuhar (1987) was obtained 20–30 minutes after the last dose, so withdrawal effects were unlikely.

Dopamine Receptor Subtypes.

There are at least two classes of dopamine receptors, which may differ in their regulation, distribution, and behavioral effects (Joyce, 1983; Stoof & Kebabian, 1984). The D1 receptor stimulates adenylate cyclase; the D2 receptor inhibits adenylate cyclase and is the dopamine receptor associated with inhibition of dopamine (by presynaptic D2 receptors), acetylcholine, and norepinephrine release in various brain regions (Joyce, 1983). So-called D3 and D4 receptors may exist as distinct entities or may represent conformations of D1 and D2 receptors (Stoof & Kebabian, 1984). Activation of these receptors has different neuroendocrine and behavioral effects in some systems (Stoof & Kebabian, 1984) but similar and perhaps synergistic effects in others (Arndt, 1985).

Relatively little is known about the role of specific dopamine receptor subtypes in effects of acute or chronic cocaine. As noted above, mesocortical D2 receptors seem to be involved in cocaine self-administration, at least in naive animals. Otherwise, there is little information about behavioral effects of these receptors outside the nigrostriatal system. Certain differences in their regulation may be relevant to chronic effects of cocaine. Receptor blockade with chronic neuroleptic treatment increases the number of D2, but not D1, receptors in the corpus striatum (MacKenzie & Zigmond, 1985). Tassin et al. (1986) reported that the development of D1 receptor supersensitivity after denervation of the prefrontal cortex depended on intact noradrenergic function. This further underscores the importance of norepinephrine in chronic effects of cocaine. As previously discussed, chronic cocaine appears to have region-specific effects on D2 receptor binding (Goeders & Kuhar, 1987), but no data on D1 binding have been reported. Cocaine reinforcement appears to involve D2 receptors, with the role of D1 receptors not established; discrimination of cocaine appears to require both types (Woolverton & Kleven, 1988; Woolverton & Virus, 1989).

Possible Neurotoxic Effects.

Treatment with high doses of methamphetamine can produce the neurotoxin 6-hydroxydopamine due to oxidation of the increased intrasynaptic dopamine (Seiden & Vosmer, 1984), and 6-hydroxydopamine can cause the degeneration of dopaminergic and noradrenergic neurons. In general, ascorbic acid may be released with dopamine as possible protection against oxidation (Louilot et al., 1985) although the actual role of the ascorbic acid is not known (Rebec et al., 1985). It is also not known whether cocaine treatment can result in the release of amounts of dopamine sufficient to produce 6-hydroxydopamine. Kleven et al. (1988) reported that levels of monoamines or their metabolites were not decreased three weeks after chronic cocaine treatment, suggesting that neuronal degeneration did not occur. Karoum et al. (1988), however, found long-lasting decreases in excretion of dopamine and its metabolites after one week or more of treatment with cocaine. Cocaine at up to 450 mg/kgld was reported not to cause degeneration (Ryan et al., 1988)

Relationship to Behavioral Adaptations to Cocaine: Tolerance, "Reverse Tolerance" (Supersensitivity), and Withdrawal

Long-term behavioral effects of cocaine have been interpreted in terms of dopamine depletion (Dackis & Gold, 1985). This model cannot account for all effects of long-term cocaine use (Dworkin &

Smith, 1986) and it is only partially consistent with the reported effects on receptor binding (Goeders & Kuhar, 1987) and dopamine storage. It can, however, explain many of the behavioral characteristics of repeated cocaine use in a parsimonious manner. In brief, the model is as follows:

1. Initial tolerance, that is, increased drug requirement for a given effect, may be an early result of dopamine depletion and consequent decreased release of dopamine. Tolerance is more commonly considered to result from receptor downregulation, or desensitization of receptors or effector systems.

2. Sensitization may result from the increase in postsynaptic receptor binding, since animals treated repeatedly with cocaine or similar drugs are more sensitive to some effects of dopamine agonists (Ellinwood et al., 1973; Kilbey & Ellinwood, 1977), as well as to cocaine itself (Kalivas et al., 1988; Kilbey & Ellinwood, 1977). Some of the mechanisms of this progressive increase in sensitivity have been interpreted in terms of kindling, as described in a later section (Post et al., 1976), and may be related to the development of psychoses during chronic drug use (Ellinwood et al., 1973). Sensitization is prevented by blockade of excitatory amino acid receptors (Karler et al., 1989a).

3. Withdrawal symptoms may stem from reduced basal dopamine release combined with increased expectation of its behavioral effects. This would result in craving and in behavioral depression.

These effects are discussed in their neurobiological context by Wise in Chapter 3 and in their clinical context by Gawin and Ellinwood in Chapter 8. For the present discussion, it is important that the changes in dopaminergic function occur in the context of altered noradrenergic and serotonergic function, which would in turn influence responses to dopamine. In addition, changes in these transmitters will affect acetylcholine, which is important in mood and in cognitive performance. For these reasons, models involving a single transmitter, though heuristically useful, are inadequate to explain the acute or chronic effects of cocaine (Dworkin & Smith, 1986).

Measurement of Dopamine Release in Vivo

In general, neurochemical measures of specific aspects of transmitter regulation require the removal of tissue and subsequent processing.

Even imaging techniques generally provide data only about isolated time points. Dopamine release can be measured in vivo using in vivo microdialysis with microvoltammetry; this technique has confirmed the presence of two functional pools of dopamine in the striatum (Ewing et al., 1983). Using in vivo microdialysis, effects of acute or chronic cocaine on release of dopamine, norepinephrine, or serotonin could be measured in specific brain regions in awake, behaving rats. This method has shown that acute administration of d-amphetamine differentially affected concentrations of ascorbic acid and of the dopamine metabolite dihydroxyphenylacetic acid (DOPAC) in the striatum and olfactory tubercle (Louilot et al., 1985).

Several investigators have used in vivo dialysis to determine effects of cocaine on extracellular dopamine concentrations in freely moving rats. Cocaine increases dopamine release in nigrostriatal and mesolimbic dopamine areas (Akimoto et al., 1989; Bradberry & Roth, 1989; Carboni et al., 1989; Di Chiara & Imperato, 1988; Hernandez & Hoebel, 1988; Nicolaysen et al., 1988; Stamford et al., 1988). The nucleus accumbens is more sensitive than the corpus striatum (Carboni et al., 1989), consistent with the evidence discussed elsewhere in this chapter that the mesolimbic dopaminergic system has weaker feedback control of its activity. This increase in nucleus accumbens dopamine release is shared by other self-administered drugs (Carboni et al., 1989; Di Chiara & Imperato, 1988) and by rewarding stimuli such as food and lateral hypothalamic self-stimulation (Hernandez & Hoebel, 1988). Subchronic cocaine treatment increased cocaine-induced dopamine efflux, consistent with behavioral sensitization (Akimoto et al., 1989).

Noradrenergic Effects of Chronic Cocaine

As with dopamine, repeated treatment with cocaine appears to deplete norepinephrine. Concentration in plasma of the norepinephrine precursors tyrosine and phenylalanine and urinary excretion of its metabolite, MHPG (an approximate measure of norepinephrine turnover), are reduced (Tennant, 1985). It is important to note, however, that reduced concentrations of oxidatively deaminated metabolites such as MHPG or of the dopamine metabolite HVA are to be expected due to reduced catecholamine reuptake

(Fekete & Borsy, 1971) and do not necessarily mean functional depletion of transmitter. Reduced noradrenergic transmitter would also appear to be consistent with a report that the number of beta-noradrenergic receptors (assayed by dihydroalprenolol [DHA] binding) is increased 50% 12 hours after a single injection of 10 mg/kg cocaine and by 250% 12 hours after discontinuation of six weeks of daily administration of cocaine in the rat, with a similar increase in norepinephrine-stimulated cyclic AMP accumulation (Banerjee et al., 1979). Interpretation of these results is complicated by the possible role of cocaine withdrawal due to the long elapsed times after drug treatment: DHA binding increased steadily from 1 to 24 hours after chronic cocaine was discontinued.

NEUROPHYSIOLOGIC EFFECTS OF COCAINE: KINDLING

Kindling refers to a class of neural phenomena in which repeated low-intensity stimulation produces a progressive increase in sensitivity leading to afterdischarges and, eventually, behavioral and electrographic convulsions (Goddard et al., 1969). Effects of cocaine on kindling may provide information about its adaptive effects on neural excitability; indeed, some of cocaine's long-term effects may be related to similar phenomena (Post et al., 1976). Monoamine neurotransmitters have important roles in kindling: Norepinephrine, for example, can inhibit kindling (Ashton et al., 1980; Mohr & Corcoran, 1981). Local anesthetics also have complex effects (Babington & Wedeking, 1973). Effects of cocaine on kindling, either by transmitter or by local anesthetic mechanisms, could include (1) alteration in characteristics of kindling produced by electrical stimulation or (2) direct effects of repeated cocaine (Post et al., 1981).

Cocaine has both proconvulsant and anticonvulsant effects on kindling produced by repeated electrical stimulation of the prepyriform cortex (Russel & Stripling, 1985; Stripling & Russel, 1985). This region is of interest because it is the primary projection of the olfactory bulb, where abnormal discharges are produced by relatively low doses of cocaine (Stripling, 1982). As both cocaine and lidocaine share certain anticonvulsant effects including reduction of the duration of the kindled afterdischarge (Stripling &

Hendricks, 1981) and the duration of afterdischarge persisting beyond clonus, these effects appear to result from local anesthetic mechanisms (Russel & Stripling, 1985). The most reliable proconvulsant effect of cocaine in this system is reduction of the latency to clonus, an expression of an acceleration by cocaine of the propagation of seizure activity from the site of origin (Lesse & Collins, 1979). This effect is also similar to that of lidocaine (Stripling & Hendricks, 1981).

Reduced duration of clonus may be related to monoamines (Ashton et al., 1980; Corcoran et al., 1974), but effects of cocaine are difficult to interpret. Russel and Stripling (1985) found that cocaine reduced clonus duration, similar to the alpha-1 antagonist prazosin; the effects of these agents were additive. These effects were similar to those previously reported for alpha-2 receptor stimulation (Ashton et al., 1980), but were not blocked by the alpha-2 antagonist yohimbine (Russel & Stripling, 1985).

The progressive sensitization to behavioral effects of cocaine by repeated cocaine treatment (Stripling et al., 1976) has been compared to kindling (Post et al., 1976). Generalized convulsions produced by high doses of cocaine facilitate subsequent kindling (Kilbey et al., 1979). Although sensitization to the behavioral effects of cocaine occurs at subconvulsive doses (Post et al., 1976; Stripling & Ellinwood, 1976), sensitization to kindled seizures does not, either in the amygdala (Kilbey et al., 1979; Post et al., 1981; Rackham & Wise, 1979) or the olfactory bulb (Stripling, 1983). This suggests that the progressive behavioral sensitization to low doses of cocaine occurs by another mechanism.

Karler et al. (1989b) recently reported that, although acute cocaine had anticonvulsant effects, daily cocaine at doses causing motor hyperactivity decreased the seizure threshold to electroconvulsive shock, without causing spontaneous seizures. Rats treated with daily cocaine developed electrically kindled seizures more rapidly.

NEUROTRANSMITTER INTERACTIONS AND COCAINE

Transmitter interactions involving cocaine can be divided into interactions between transmitters affected directly by cocaine, and indirect effects of changes in these transmitters on other transmitters. These will be discussed in terms of reported effects of cocaine, and of possible involvement in cocaine effects when they have not yet been examined.

Interactions between Norepinephrine and Dopamine

Norepinephrine and dopamine are thought to have complementary neurophysiologic roles (Oades, 1985). Because cocaine affects both, interactions between these transmitters may be important in its long-term effects. Possible influences of norepinephrine on aspects of behavior that are primarily dependent on dopamine may be especially relevant to cocaine effects. Kellogg and Wennerstrom (1974) and Geyer and Segal (1974) proposed that, in intact animals, norepinephrine would inhibit behavioral actions of dopamine. Pycock et al., 1975, however, reported evidence for facilitation of dopamine effects by norepinephrine. The interactions between these transmitters may therefore depend on environmental factors (Antelman et al., 1976).

Norepinephrine-dopamine interactions, possibly influenced by environmental stress or activation, have been reported for a range of dopaminergic effects on behavior. Stereotypy, associated with activation of the nigrostriatal dopamine system, is reduced when dopamine is depleted, but is not altered if both norepinephrine and dopamine are depleted (Hollister et al., 1974). Similarly, inhibition of dopamine beta-hydroxylase, the enzyme that converts dopamine to norepinephrine, reduced methylphenidate-induced hyperactivity (Breese et al., 1975). Amphetamine-induced hyperactivity was increased by depletion of norepinephrine, decreased by depletion of dopamine, and not altered by depletion of both dopamine and norepinephrine; consistent with a possible role of stress in these effects, norepinephrine depletion did not alter spontaneous motor activity (Evetts et al., 1970). Parallel effects on shock-elicited fighting have been reported (Geyer & Segal, 1974). Perhaps most relevant to the situation with cocaine, Koob et al. (1976) reported that ipsilateral lesions of noradrenergic neurons in the locus coeruleus increased lateral hypothalamic self-stimulation.

Antelman and Caggiula (1977) have interpreted norepinephrine-dopamine interactions in a manner that might be particularly relevant to effects of cocaine. They suggest that norepinephrine modulates primarily dopaminergic effects on behavior, and that the direction of this modulation depends on the level of arousal: enhancement in states of high arousal and inhibition when arousal is lower. "Arousal" as defined by Antelman and Caggiulia has unknown neurochemical correlates, but is likely to be associated with acetylcholine (Castellani et al., 1983; Celesia & Jasper, 1963).

In addition to direct effects on both catecholamines, cocaine's effects on either may have indirect effects on the other. In the case of acute treatment, there would initially be a net increase in synaptic dopamine and norepinephrine. Increased dopamine release would reduce the firing rate of noradrenergic cells, and norepinephrine release, by binding to presynaptic dopamine receptors on noradrenergic terminals (Misu et al., 1985) as well as by direct alpha-2 agonist actions (Jackisch et al., 1985). Norepinephrine can, in turn, modulate mesolimbic dopamine release, since the beta-receptor agonist isoproterenol increases, whereas the alpha- 2 agonist clonidine decreases, depolarization-evoked dopamine release in the nucleus accumbens (Nurse et al., 1984).

Long-term effects would depend on the relative responses of noradrenergic and dopaminergic systems to repeated stimulation. Dopamine appears more sensitive to precursor supply (Milner & Wurtman, 1986), although evidence cited above indicates that both amines may be depleted during chronic cocaine (Banerjee et al., 1979; Taylor et al., 1979), at least in some brain regions (Goeders & Kuhar, 1987). Relative sparing of the labile (alpha-methylparatyrosine-sensitive) pool of dopamine, combined with the relative lack of distinguishable pools of norepinephrine (Lawson- Wendling et al., 1981), might alter the balance between dopaminergic and noradrenergic effects during repeated cocaine treatment. This has never been examined directly, however.

In summary, hypotheses of combined dopamine-norepinephrine effects of chronic cocaine could include the following: (1) Depletion of norepinephrine during chronic cocaine would reduce effects of dopamine depletion; (2) in the presence of relatively high stress or arousal, dopaminergic effects of cocaine, including its reward effects, would be facilitated by norepinephrine; and (3) the level of environmental arousal, and/or manipulation of cholinergic systems, would be expected to have an important influence on the behavioral effectiveness of repeated cocaine, and possibly on cocaine withdrawal. Testing of these and other hypotheses will require more information about the transmitter effects of single doses of cocaine in animals or humans who have been chronically treated with the drug.

Serotonin-norepinephrine Interactions.

There is little information about the effects of chronic cocaine on serotonergic receptors. Long-term depletion of serotonin could have important effects on adaptations in other monoamines. For example, serotonin depletion increases the number of beta-receptors in the rat hippocampus and cerebral cortex (Manier et al., 1987) and prevents the decrease in beta-receptor binding after chronic desipramine (Manier et al., 1987; Stockmeier et al., 1985). Conversely, beta-noradrenergic receptor stimulation increases serotonin-2 (but not serotonin-1) receptor binding (Scott & Crews, 1985) and inhibition of norepinephrine release with low-dose clonidine increases tryptophan hydroxylase activity (Weekley et al., 1985). If long-term cocaine treatment depletes serotonin, it could therefore prevent receptor adaptations to repeated noradrenergic stimulation by acute cocaine; in fact, serotonin depletion may contribute to the increase in beta-receptor binding during chronic cocaine administration reported by Banerjee et al. (1979). Failure of beta-receptors to adapt to increased norepinephrine would enhance noradrenergic toxicity during cocaine use.

Serotonin-dopamine Interactions.

Serotonergic and dopaminergic activity appear to be regulated in parallel (Bowers, 1972), with serotonin opposing self-administration of stimulant drugs (Ritz & Kuhar, 1989). Dopamine generally seems to increase behavior related to aggression, whereas serotonin inhibits it (Benkert et al., 1973; Pradhan, 1974). Low serotonin function in humans may be associated with increased aggression (Brown et al., 1979; Muhlbauer, 1985). In general, the aggressive behavior that would be associated with increased dopamine would be inhibited by the accompanying increase in serotonin. Cocaine,

however, increases dopaminergic transmission while inhibiting serotonin synthesis, so the balancing inhibitory effect of serotonin on
aggression would be missing. Cocaine therefore has at least the potential of increasing aggression more than other stimulants that increase both dopamine and serotonin.

Role of Peptides Released with Monoamines

Cholecystokinin is released with dopamine and amplifies its behavioral effects in the nucleus accumbens, but not in the caudate
(Crawley et al., 1984). In addition, norepinephrine (neuropeptide
Y) and serotonin are coreleased with neuropeptides, at least in some
of their terminals (Krieger, 1983). The effects of acute or chronic
cocaine on release or function of these peptides are not known.

Interactions between Catecholamines and Acetylcholine

Dopamine inhibits release of acetylcholine via presynaptic D2 receptors on cholinergic terminals (Baud et al., 1985; Gilad et al.,
1986; Hoffmann & Cubeddu, 1984; Wong et al., 1983). In turn,
acetylcholine (possibly via M2 muscarinic receptors) apparently increases dopamine release in the corpus striatum (Potter et al., 1985;
Wilson et al., 1977). Acetylcholine, however, does not appear to
affect mesolimbic dopamine release (Consolo et al., 1977). Long-
term dopaminergic treatments have effects opposite to those of
acute treatment: Haloperidol increased evoked acetylcholine release,
whereas bromocriptine reduced it (Cubeddu et al., 1983). Cocaine
itself has been reported to reduce acetylcholine release in vitro by
several mechanisms: increased dopamine release, direct dopaminergic agonist effects (at 10 μM concentrations) and local anesthetic effects on Na^+ channels (Hoffmann et al., 1986).

The effects of long-term or repeated cocaine treatment on cholinergic function are unknown. Cholinergic effects may be important in both cognitive and behavioral (Vrijmoed-de Vries & Cools,
1985) effects of cocaine. Blockage of cholinergic receptors reduces
the intravenous self-administration of cocaine (Wilson & Schuster,
1973; Woolverton & Goldberg, 1984). Acetylcholine also influences

the development of cocaine-induced seizures, by increasing preco-caine arousal and inhibiting seizure development (Castellani et al., 1983).

Despite the evidence suggesting inhibition of acetylcholine re-lease, acute cocaine has been reported to increase acetylcholine turn-over in the hippocampus (Robinson & Hambrecht, 1988). There is a preliminary report that cocaine treatment also caused a cholinergically mediated behavioral and EEG arousal (Yabase et al., 1989).

Norepinephrine also reduces acetylcholine release (Wetzel & Brown, 1985). Treatment with d-amphetamine appears to reduce acetylcholine turnover via a noradrenergic mechanism, since the ef-fect is prevented by lesion of the ventral noradrenergic bundle (Robinson, 1986).

Gamma-aminobutyric acid (GABA) has important interactions with dopamine and, like acetylcholine, is involved in a negative feedback loop with the nigrostriatal system (Gale & Casu, 1981). We know of no information about long-term effects of cocaine on GABAergic function.

PROBLEMS IN INTERPRETATION OF COCAINE EFFECTS

Although information is available to answer some of the questions raised at the beginning of this chapter, others remain unresolved. A brief summary of the state of these problems follows:

1. Although cocaine is only a modestly effective monoamine re-uptake blocker in vitro, effective concentrations are readily attained in vivo. Differences between cocaine and other stimulants or reup-take blockers may arise because of its differential effects: sparing of the labile pool of dopamine; local anesthetic effect; inhibition of tryptophan transport; relative lack of effects on postsynaptic monoaminergic receptors; and equipotent blockage of dopamine, norepinephrine, and serotonin reuptake rather than relative specific-ity for a single amine.

2. It may appear paradoxical that, in the context of long-term treatment that depletes dopamine in at least some brain regions, acute cocaine continues to produce effects consistent with surges of increased dopamine. Although cocaine depletes the stable, reserpine-sensitive pool of dopamine, it spares the labile, alpha-methyltyrosine-sensitive pool. Cocaine can also act intrasynaptically to increase dopamine synthesis. In addition, receptor and uptake studies suggest that the net effect of cocaine on synaptic dopamine varies among brain regions, with possible depletion in the mesolimbic and mesocortical but not the nigrostriatal systems. This difference may be related to better developed feedback regulation of nigrostriatal dopaminergic function.

3. In terms of adaptations in other transmitters during chronic cocaine, relatively little is known about receptor or second messenger alterations, especially in different brain regions or functional systems (i.e., locus coeruleus vs. lateral tegmental noradrenergic systems). In general, there is relatively little information about the noradrenergic and serotonergic effects of cocaine.

Data suggest strongly that acetylcholine is involved in the behavioral and cognitive effects of cocaine, but there is little information about the cholinergic effects of chronic cocaine. Cholinergic deficits could contribute to cognitive impairments that develop during chronic cocaine use.

DISCUSSION AND CONCLUSIONS

The synaptic effects of cocaine and the adaptations to them can be summarized as follows:

1. The reward and self-administration effects of cocaine are associated primarily with dopaminergic effects, largely in the prefrontal cortex.

2. Monoamine reuptake and Na^+ channel blockade have similar concentration requirements, falling within those readily reached in vivo. Although the role of Na^+ channel blockade in behavior is not clear, it seems especially important in the acute noradrenergic effects.

3. Cocaine can act intrasynaptically to increase dopamine synthesis, in addition to its inhibition of reuptake.

4. Cocaine binding sites are associated at least with dopamine and serotonin reuptake sites. Little is known about their regulation, other than their destruction by selective neurotoxins.

5. In terms of transmitter synthesis and neuronal activity, acute treatment in vivo increases dopamine synthesis, reduces serotonin synthesis, and reduces firing rates of presynaptic dopaminergic, noradrenergic, and serotonergic cells.

6. Repeated cocaine administration was reported to increase noradrenergic and dopaminergic receptor binding under conditions that might have been associated with cocaine withdrawal. More recent studies reported increased dopaminergic receptor binding in the nucleus accumbens and decreased receptor binding in the caudate. Long-term dopaminergic effects may therefore differ for the mesolimbic and nigrostriatal systems: The mesolimbic/mesocortical system, with its relative lack of autoreceptors, may be more sensitive to dopamine depletion.

7. Cocaine has complicated effects on limbic kindled seizures, including proconvulsant and anticonvulsant effects based on both Na^+ channel blockade and monoamine reuptake inhibition. Progressive behavioral sensitization to subconvulsant doses of cocaine does not appear directly related to kindling.

8. Effects on norepinephrine-dopaminergic interactions, and on peptides coreleased with monoamines, are unknown. Cocaine decreases acetylcholine release in vitro and there is an important cholinergic-dopaminergic feedback loop, but cocaine effects in vivo are not known.

9. The relative inhibition of serotonergic transmission by cocaine may have a major impact on its behavioral and adaptive effects, including (a) disinhibition of aggression and (b) impairment of noradrenergic receptor downregulation in response to norephinephrine. This would lead in turn to (c) increased sensitivity to aggression stimulated by dopamine and (d) toxic effects of surges of NE release in the face of receptor supersensitivity. The last may be an important contributor to deadly noradrenergic toxic episodes in cocaine users.

The results summarized in this chapter show that there is much to be learned about the neural mechanisms that produce cocaine's acute and chronic effects. These are bound up intimately with regulation of vital reward systems in the brain. Investigation of these mechanisms will therefore provide, in addition to information about a major drug of abuse, important knowledge about basic functions of the brain.

REFERENCES

Akimoto, K., Hamamura, T. & Ot-suki, S. (1989) Subchronic cocaine treatment enhances cocaine-induced dopamine efflux, studied by in vivo intracerebral dialysis. *Brain Res.* 490:339–344.

Antelman, S. M. & Caggiula, A. R. (1977) Norepinephrine-dopamine interactions and behavior. *Science* 195:646–653.

Antelman, S. M., Rowland, N. E. & Fisher, A. S. (1976) Stress-related recovery from lateral hypothalamic aphasia. *Brain Res.* 102:346–350.

Arndt, J. (1985) Hyperactivity induced by stimulation of separate dopamine D-1 and D-2 receptors in rats with bilateral 6-OHDA lesions. *Life Sci.* 37:717–723.

Ashton, D., Leysen, J. E. & Wauquier, A. (1980) Neurotransmitters and receptor binding in amygdaloid kindled rats: Serotonergic and noradrenergic modulatory effects. *Life Sci.* 27:1547–1556.

Aston-Jones, S., Aston-Jones, G. & Koob, G. F. (1984) Cocaine antagonizes anxiolytic effects of ethanol. *Psychopharmacology* 84:28–31.

Babington, R. G. & Wedeking, P. W. (1973) The pharmacology of seizures induced by sensitization with low intensity brain stimulation. *Pharmacol. Biochem. Behav.* 1:461–467.

Bagchie, S. P. (1985) Cocaine and phencyclidine. Heterogenous dopaminergic interactions with tetrabenazine. *Neuropharmacology* 24:37–41.

Bagchie, S. P. & Reilly, M. A. (1983) Intraneuronal dopaminergic action of cocaine and some of its metabolites and analogs. *Neuropharmacology* 22:1289–1295.

Bagchie, S. P., Smith, T. M. & Bagchie, P. (1980) Divergent reserpine effects on amfonelic acid and amphetamine stimulation of synaptosomal dopamine formation from phenylalanine. *Biochem. Pharmacol.* 29:2957–1602.

Banerjee, D. K., Lutz, R. A., Levine, M. A., Rodbard, D. & Pollard, H. B. (1987) Uptake of norepinephrine and related catecholamines by cultured chromaffin cells: Characterization of cocaine-sensitive and -insensitive plasma membrane transport sites. *Proc. Nat. Acad. Sci. USA* 84:1749–1753.

Banerjee, S. P., Sharma, V. K., Kung-Cheung, L., Chanda, S. K. & Riggi, S. K. (1979) Cocaine and d-amphetamine induced changes in central beta-adrenoceptor sensitivity: Effects of acute and chronic drug treatment. *Brain Res.* 175:119–130.

Bannon, M. J., Michaud, R. L. & Roth, R. H. (1981) Mesocortical dopamine neurons. Lack of autoreceptors modulating dopamine synthesis. *Mol. Pharmacol.* 19:270–275.

Bannon, M. J. & Roth, R. H. (1983) Pharmacology of mesocortical dopamine neurons. *Pharmacol. Rev.* 35:53–68.

Baud, P., Arbilla, S. & Langer, S. Z. (1985) Inhibition of the electrically evoked release of [^{3}H]acetylcholine in rat striatal slices: An experimental model for drugs that enhance dopaminergic neurotransmission. *J. Neurochem.* 44:331–337.

Benkert, O., Renz, A. & Matussek, N. (1973) Dopamine, noradrenaline, and 5-hydroxytryptamine in relation to motor activity, fighting, and mounting behavior. *Neuropharmacology* 12:187–193.

Bowers, M. B., Jr. (1972) Clinical measurement of central dopamine and serotonin metabolism: Reliability and interpretation of cerebrospinal fluid monoamine measures. *Neuropharmacology* 11:101–111.

Bradberry, C. W. & Roth, R. H. (1989) Cocaine increases extracellular dopamine in rat nucleus accumbens and ventral tegmental area as shown by in vivo microdialysis. *Neurosci. Lett.* 103: 97–102.

Breese, G. R., Casper, G. R. & Hollister, A. S. (1975) Involvement of brain monoamines in the stimulant and paradoxical inhibitory effect of methylphenidate. *Psychopharmacologia* 44:5–10.

Brown, G. L., Goodwin, F. K., Ballenger, J. C., Goyer, P. F. & Major, L. F. (1979) Aggression in humans correlates with cerebrospinal fluid amine levels. *Psychiat. Res.* 1:131–139.

Carboni, E., Imperato, A., Perezzani, L. & Di Chiara, G. (1989) Amphetamine, cocaine, phencyclidine, and nomifensine increase extracellular dopamine concentrations preferentially in nucleus accumbens of freely moving rats. *Neuroscience* 28:653–661.

Castellani, S., Ellinwood, E. H., Jr., Kilbey, M. M. & Petrie, W. M. (1983) Cholinergic effects on arousal and cocaine-induced olfactory-amygdala spindling and seizures in rats. *Physiol. Behav.* 31:461–466.

Celesia, C. G. & Jasper, H. H. (1963) Acetylcholine release from cerebral cortex in relation to state of activation. *Neurology* 16:1053–1063.

Chapman, D. & Hayward, J. A. (1985) New biophysical techniques and their application to the study of membranes. *Biochem. J.* 228:281–295.

Clark, D., Hjorth, S. & Carlsson, A. (1985a) Dopamine receptor agonists: Mechanisms underlying autoreceptor selectivity. II. Theoretical considerations. *J. Neural Trans.* 62:171–207.

Clark, D., Hjorth, S. & Carlsson, A. (1985b) Dopamine receptor agonists: Mechanisms underlying autoreceptor selectivity. I. Review of the evidence. *J. Neural Trans.* 62:1–52.

Consolo, S., Landinsky, H., Bianchi, S. & Ghezzi, D. (1977) Apparent lack of a dopaminergic-cholinergic link in the rat nucleus accumbens septituberculum olfactorium. *Brain Res.* 135:255–263.

Corcoran, M. E., Fibiger, H. C., McCaughran, J. A. & Wada, J. A. (1974) Potentiation of amygdaloid kindling and metrazole-induced seizures by 6-hydroxydopamine in rats. *Exp. Neurol.* 45:118–133.

Crawley, J. N., Hommer, D. W. & Skirboll, L. R. (1984) Behavioral and neurophysiological evidence for a facilitatory interaction between co-existing transmitters: Cholecystokinin and dopamine. *Neurochem. Int.* 6:755–760.

Creese, I. & Iversen, S. D. (1975) The pharmacological and anatomical substrates of the amphetamine response in the rat. *Brain Res.* 83:419–436.

Cregler, L. L. & Mark, H. (1986) Medical complications of cocaine abuse. *N. Engl. J. Med.* 315:1495–1500.

Cubeddu, L. X., Hoffmann, I. S., James, M. K. & Niedzwiecki, D. M. (1983) Changes in the sensitivity to apomorphine of dopamine receptors modulating dopamine and acetylocholine release after chronic treatment with bromocriptine or haloperidol. *J. Pharmacol. Exp. Ther.* 226:680–685.

Cunningham, K. A. & Lakoski, J. M. (1988) Electrophysiological effects of cocaine and procaine on dorsal raphe serotonin neurons. *Eur. J. Pharmacol.* 148:457–462.

Dackis, C. A. & Gold, M. S. (1985) New concepts in cocaine addiction: The dopamine depletion hypothesis. *Neurosci. Biobehav. Rev.* 9:469–477.

Dackis, C. A., Gold, M. S. & Estroff, T. W. (1984) Hyperprolactinemia in cocaine abuse. *Soc. Neurosci. Abstr.* 10:1099.

Dart, A. M., Dietz, R., Kubler, W., Schomig, A. & Strasser, R. (1983) Effects of cocaine and desipramine on the neurally evoked overflow of endogenous noradrenaline from the rat heart. *Br. J. Pharmacol.* 79:71–74.

Davis, M. (1985) Cocaine: Excitatory effects on sensorimotor reactivity measured with acoustic startle. *Psychopharmacology* 86:31–36.

Demarest, K. T. & Moore, K. E. (1979) Comparison of dopamine synthesis regulation in the terminals of nigrostriatal, mesolimbic, tuberoinfundibular and tuberohypophyseal neurons. *J. Neural. Trans.* 46:263–277.

Di Chiara, G. & Imperato, A. (1988) Drugs abused by humans increase synaptic dopamine concentrations in the mesolimbic system of freely moving rats. *Proc. Nat. Acad. Sci. USA* 85:5274–5278.

DiGiulio, A. M., Groppetti, A. & Cattabeni, F. (1978) Significance of dopamine metabolites in the evaluation of drugs acting on dopaminergic neurons. *Eur. J. Pharmacol.* 52:201–207.

Dworkin, S. I. & Smith, J. E. (1986) Neurobiological aspects of drug-seeking behaviors. In: Dews, P. B., Thompson, T. & Barrett, J. E. (Eds.), *Neurobehavioral pharmacology: Advances in behavioral pharmacology, vol. 6.* Hillsdale, N.J.: Lawrence Erlbaum, 1–43.

Einhorn, L. C., Johansen, P. A. & White, F. J. (1988) Electrophysiological effects of cocaine in the mesoaccumbens dopamine system: Studies in the ventral tegmental area. *J. Neurosci.* 8:100–112.

Ellinwood, E. H., Sudilovsky, A. & Nelson, L. M. (1973) Evolving behavior in the clinical and experimental amphetamine (model) psychosis. *Am. J. Psychiat.* 130:1088–1093.

El Mestikawy, S., Glowinski, J. & Hamon, M. (1986) Presynaptic dopamine autoreceptors control tyrosine hydroxylase activation in depolarized striatal dopaminergic terminals. *J. Neurochem.* 46:12–22.

Evetts, K. D., Uretsky, N. J., Iversen, L. L. & Iversen, S. D. (1970) Effects of 6-hydroxydopamine on CNS catecholamines, spontaneous motor activity, and amphetamine-induced hyperactivity in the rat. *Nature* 225:961–962.

Ewing, A.G., Bigelow, J. C. & Wrightman, R. M. (1983) Direct in vivo monitoring of dopamine released from two striatal compartments in the rat. *Science* 221:169–171.

Fekete, M. & Borsy, J. (1971) Chlorpromazine-cocaine antagonism: Its relation to changes of dopamine metabolism in the brain. *Eur. J. Pharmacol.* 16:171–175.

Fozard, J. R., Mobarok, A.T.M. & Newgrosh, G. (1979) Blockade of serotonin receptors on automatic neurons by (−) cocaine and some related compounds. *Eur. J. Pharmacol.* 59:195–210.

Freud, S. (1884) Uber Coca. *Centralblatt f. d. ges. Therap.* 2:289–314.

Friedman, E., Gershon, S. & Rotrosen, J. (1975) Effects of acute cocaine treatment on the turnover of 5-hydroxytryptamine in rat brain. *Br. J. Pharmacol.* 54:61–64.

Fuder, H., Bath, F., Weibelt, H. & Muscholl, E. (1984) Autoinhibition of adrenaline release from the rat heart as a function of the biophase concentration. Effects of exogenous alpha-adrenoceptor agonists, cocaine, and perfusion rate. *Naunyn-Schmiedeberg's Arch. Pharmacol.* 325:25–33.

Gale, K. & Casu, M. (1981) Dynamic utilization of GABA in substantia nigra: Regulation by dopamine and GABA in the striatum and its clinical and biochemical implications. *Mol. Cell. Biochem.* 39:369–405.

Gawin, F. H. (1986) Neuroleptic reduction of cocaine-induced paranoia but not euphoria? *Psychopharmacology* 90:142–143.

Geyer, M. A. & Segal, D. S. (1974) Shock-induced aggression: Opposite effects of intraventricularly infused dopamine and norepinephrine. *Behav. Biol.* 10:99–104.

Giannini, A. J., Malone, D. A., Loiselle, R. H. & Price, W. A. (1987) Blunting of TSH response to TRH in chronic cocaine and phencyclidine abusers. *J. Clin. Psychiat.* 48:25–26.

Gilad, G. M., Gilad, V. H. & Rabey, J. M. (1986) Dopaminergic modulation of the septo-hippocampal cholinergic system activity under stress. *Life Sci.* 39:2387–2393.

Goddard, G. V., McIntyre, D. C. & Leech, C. K. (1969) A permanent change in brain function resulting from daily electrical stimulation. *Exp. Neurol.* 25:295–330.

Goeders, N. E. & Kuhar, M. J. (1987) Chronic cocaine induces opposite changes in dopamine receptors in the striatum and nucleus accumbens. *Alcohol Drug Res.* 7:207–216.

Goeders, N. E. & Smith, J. E. (1983) Cortical dopaminergic involvement in cocaine reinforcement. *Science* 221:773–775.

Goeders, N. E. & Smith, J. E. (1986) Reinforcing properties of cocaine in the medial prefrontal cortex: Primary action on presynaptic dopaminergic terminals. *Pharmacol. Biochem. Behav.* 25:191–199.

Hadfield, M. G. & Nugent, E. A. (1983) Cocaine: Comparative effect on dopamine uptake in extrapyramidal and limbic systems. *Biochem. Pharmacol.* 32:744–746.

Halbreich, U., Sachar, E. J. & Asnis, G. M. (1981) The prolactin response to intravenous dextroamphetamine in normal young men and postmenopausal women. *Life Sci.* 28:2337–2342.

Hernandez, L. & Hoebel, B. G. (1988) Food reward and cocaine increase extracellular dopamine in the nucleus accumbens as measured by microdialysis. *Life Sci.* 42:1705–1712.

Hoffman, I. S. & Cubeddu, L. X. (1984) Differential effects of bromocriptine on dopamine and acetylcholine release modulatory receptors. *J. Neurochem.* 42:278–282.

Hoffmann, I. S., Talmaciu, R. K., & Cubeddu, L. X. (1986) Interactions between endogenous dopamine and dopamine agonists at release modulatory receptors: Multiple effects of neuronal uptake inhibitors on transmitter release. *J. Pharmacol. Exp. Ther.* 238:437–446.

Hollister, A. S., Breese, G. R. & Casper, B. R. (1974) Comparison of tyrosine hydroxylase and dopamine beta-hydroxylase inhibition with the effects of various 6-hydroxydopamine treatments on d-amphetamine induced motor activity. *Psychopharmacologia* 36:1–16.

Holmstedt, B. & Fregda, A. (1981) Sundry episodes in the history of coca and cocaine. *J. Ethnopharmacol.* 3:113–147.

Jackson, I. (1982) Thyrotropin-releasing hormone. *N. Engl. J. Med.* 306:145–155.

Jackisch, R., Moll, S., Feuerstein, T. J. & Hertting, G. (1985) Dopaminergic modulation of hippocampal noradrenaline release. Evidence for alpha-2 antagonistic effects of some dopamine receptor agonists and antagonists. *Naunyn-Schmiedeberg's Arch. Pharmacol.* 330: 105–115.

Joyce, J. N. (1983) Multiple dopamine receptors and behavior. *Neurosci. Biobehav. Rev.* 7:227–256.

Kalivas, P. W., Duffy, P., DuMars, L. A. & Skinner, C. (1988) Behavioral and neurochemical effects of acute and daily cocaine administration in rats. *J. Pharmacol. Exp. Ther.* 245:485–492.

Karler, R., Calder, L. D., Chaudry, I. A. & Turkanis, S. A. (1989a) Blockade of "reverse tolerance" to cocaine and amphetamine by MK-801. *Life Sci.* 45:599–606.

Karler, R., Petty, C., Calder, L. & Turkanis, S. A. (1989b) Proconvulsant and anticonvulsant effects in mice of acute and chronic treatment with cocaine. *Neuropharmacology* 28:709–714.

Karoum, F., Fawcett, R. W. & Wyatt, R. J. (1988) Chronic cocaine effects on peripheral biogenic amines: A longterm reduction in peripheral dopamine and phenylethylamine production. *Eur. J. Pharmacol.* 148:381–388.

Kellogg, C. & Wennerstrom, G. (1974) An ontogenic study on the effect of catecholamine receptor stimulating agents on the turnover of noradrenaline and dopamine in the brain. *Brain Res.* 79:451–464.

Kennedy, L. T. & Hanbauer, I. (1983) Sodium-sensitive cocaine binding to rat striatal membrane: Possible relationship to dopamine uptake sites. *J. Neurochem.* 41:172–178.

Kilbey, M. M. & Ellinwood, E. H. (1977) Reverse tolerance to stimulant-induced abnormal behavior. *Life Sci.* 20:1063–1076.

Kilbey, M. M., Ellinwood, E. H., Jr. & Easler, M. E. (1979) The effects of chronic cocaine pretreatment on kindled seizures and behavioral stereotypes. *Exp. Neurol.* 64:306–314.

Kleven, M. S., Woolverton, W. L. & Seiden, L. S. (1988) Lack of longterm monoamine depletions following repeated or continuous exposure to cocaine. *Brain Res. Bull.* 21:233–237.

Knapp, S. & Mandell, A. J. (1972) Narcotic drugs: Effects on serotonin biosynthetic systems of the brain. *Science* 177:1209–1211.

Koob, G. F., Balcomb, G. J. & Meyerhoff, J. L. (1976) Increases in intracranial self-stimulation in the posterior hypothalamus following unilateral lesions in the locus coeruleus. *Brain Res.* 101:554–560.

Kornhuber, J. & Kornhuber, M. E. (1986) Presynaptic modulation of cortical input to the striatum. *Life Sci.* 39: 669–674.

Krieger, D. T. (1983) Brain peptides: What, where and why? *Science* 222:975–985.

Kuhn, C. M., Vogel, R. A. & Mailman, R. B. (1981) Effect of 5,7-dihydroxytryptamine on central serotonergic regulation of prolactin release and behavior in rats. *Psychopharmacology* 73: 1088–1093.

Lane, J. D., Sands, M. P., Co., C., Cherek, D. R. & Smith, J. E. (1982) Monoamine turnover in discrete rat brain regions is correlated with conditioned emotional response and with its conditioning history. *Brain Res.* 240:95–108.

Lawson-Wendling, K. L., Demarest, K. T. & Moore, K. E. (1981) Differential effects of (+)-amphetamine, methylphenidate, and amfonelic acid on catecholamine synthesis in selected regions of the rat brain. *J. Pharm. Pharmacol.* 33:803–804.

Lazar, M. A., Mefford, I. N. & Barchas, J. D. (1982) Tyrosine hydroxylase activation. Comparison of in vitro phosphorylation and in vivo administration of haloperidol. *Biochem. Pharmacol.* 31:2599–2607.

Lesse, H. & Collins, J. P. (1979) Effects of cocaine on propagation of limbic seizure activity. *Pharmacol. Biochem. Behav.* 11:689–694.

Lew, M. J. & Angus, J. A. (1983) Disadvantages of cocaine as a neuronal uptake blocking agent: Comparison with desipramine in guinea-pig right atrium. *J. Auton. Pharmacol.* 3:61–71.

Loosen, P. T. & Prange, A. J., Jr. (1982) The serum thyrotropin response to thyrotropin-releasing hormone in psychiatric patients: A review. *Am. J. Psychiat.* 139:405–416.

Louilot, A., Gonon, F., Buda, M., Simon, H., Le Moal, M. & Pujol, J. F. (1985) Effects of D- and L-amphetamine on dopamine metabolism and ascorbic acid levels in nucleus accumbens and olfactory tubercle as studied by in vivo differential pulse voltammetry. *Brain Res.* 336:253–263.

MacKenzie, R. G. & Zigmond, M. J. (1985) Chronic neuroleptic treatment increases D-2 but not D-1 receptors in rat striatum. *Eur. J. Pharmacol.* 113:159–165.

Manier, D. H., Gillespie, D. D., Sanders-Bush, E. & Sulser, F. (1987) The serotonin/noradrenaline link in brain. I. The role of noradrenaline and serotonin in the regulation of density and function of beta adrenoceptors and its alteration by desipramine. *Naunyn-Schmiedeberg's Arch. Pharmacol.* 335:109–114.

Martin-Iversen, M. T., Szostak, C.

& Fibiger, H. C. (1986) 6-hydroxydopamine lesions of the medial prefrontal cortex fail to influence intravenous self-administration of cocaine. *Psychopharmacology* 88:310–314.

Mathews, J. C. & Collins, A. (1983) Interactions of cocaine and cocaine congeners with sodium channels. *Biochem. Pharmacol.* 32:455–460.

McLeod, R. M. & Login, I. (1976) Control of prolactin secretion by the hypothalamic catecholamines. *Adv. Sex Horm. Res.* 2:211–231.

McMillan, B. A. (1982) Striatal synaptosomal tyrosine hydroxylase activity. A model system for study of presynaptic dopamine receptors. *Biochem. Pharmacol.* 31:2643–2647.

Milner, J. D. & Wurtman, R. J. (1985) Tyrosine availability determines stimulus-evoked dopamine release from rat striatal slices. *Neurosci. Let.* 59:215–220.

Milner, J. D. & Wurtman, R. J. (1986) Catecholamine synthesis: Physiological coupling to precursor supply. *Biochem. Pharmacol.* 35:875–881.

Missale, C., Castelletti, L., Govoni, S., Spano, P. F., Trabucchi, M. & Hanbauer, I. (1985) Dopamine uptake is differentially regulated in rat striatum and nucleus accumbens. *J. Neurochem.* 45:51–56.

Misu, Y., Goshima, Y., Ueda, H. & Kubo, T. (1985) Presynaptic inhibitory dopamine receptors on noradrenergic nerve terminals: Analysis of biphasic actions of dopamine and apomorphine on the release of endogenous norepinephrine in rat hypothalamic slices. *J. Pharmacol. Exp. Ther.* 235:771–777.

Mohr, E. & Corcoran, M. E. (1981) Depletion of noradrenaline and amygdaloid kindling. *Exp. Neurol.* 72:507–511.

Moore, R. Y. & Bloom, F. E. (1978) Central catecholamine neuron systems: Anatomy and physiology of dopamine systems. *Ann. Rev. Neurosci.* 1:129–169.

Morency, M. & Beninger, R. J. (1986) Dopaminergic substrates of cocaine-induced place conditioning. *Brain Res.* 399:33–41.

Morency, M. A., Stewart, R. J. & Beninger, R. J. (1987) Circling behavior following unilateral microinjections of cocaine into the medial prefontal cortex: Dopaminergic or local anesthetic effect? *J. Neurosci.* 7:812–818.

Muhlbauer, H. D. (1985) Human aggression and the role of central serotonin. *Pharmacopsychiat.* 18:218–221.

Nicolaysen, L. C., Pan, H. T. & Justice, J. B., Jr. (1988) Extracellular cocaine and dopamine concentrations are linearly correlated in rat striatum. *Brain Res.* 456:317–323.

Nurse, B., Russel, V. A. & Taljaard, J.J.F. (1984) Alpha-2 and beta-adrenoceptor agonists modulate [3H]dopamine release from rat nucleus accumbens slices: Implications for research into depression. *Neurochem. Res.* 9:1231–1238.

Oades, R. D. (1985) The role of noradrenaline in tuning and dopamine in switching between signals in the CNS. *Neurosci. Biobehav. Rev.* 9:261–282.

Pelayo, F., Dubocovich, M. L. & Langer, S. Z. (1980) Inhibition of neuronal uptake reduces the presynaptic effect of clonidine but not of alpha-methylnorepinephrine on the stimulus-evoked release of 3H-norepinephrine from rat occipital cortex slices. *Eur. J. Pharmacol.* 64:143–155.

Pettit, W. O., Ettenberg, A., Bloom, F. E. & Koob, G. F. (1984) Destruction of dopamine in the nucleus accumbens selectively attenuates cocaine but not heroin self-administration in rats. *Psychopharmacology* 84:167–173.

Pimoule, C., Schoemaker, H., Javoy-Agid, F., Scatton, B. & Agid, Y. (1983) Decrease in [3H]cocaine binding to the dopamine transporter in Parkinson's disease. *Eur. J. Pharmacol.* 95:145–146.

Pitts, D. K. & Marwah, J. (1986) Effects of cocaine on the electrical activity of single noradrenergic neurons from locus coeruleus. *Life Sci.* 38:1229–1234.

Pitts, D. K. & Marwah, J. (1987) Cocaine modulation of central monoamine neurotransmission. *Pharmacol. Biochem. Behav.* 26:453–461.

Post, R. M., Kopanda, R. T. & Black, K. E. (1976) Progressive effects of cocaine on behavior and central amine metabolism in rhesus monkeys: Relationship to kindling and psychosis. *Biol. Psychiat.* 11:403–419.

Post, R. M., Squillace, K. M., Pert, A. & Sass, W. (1981) The effect of amygdala kindling on spontaneous and cocaine-induced motor activity and lidocaine seizures. *Psychopharmacology* 72: 189–196.

Potter, P. E., Hadjiconstantinou, M., Rubenstein, J. S. & Neff, N. (1985) Chronic treatment with diisopropyl-fluorophosphate increases dopamine turnover in the striatum of the rat. *Eur. J. Pharmacol.* 106:607–611.

Pradhan, S. (1983) Effect of cocaine on rat brain enzymes. *Arch. Int. Pharmacodyn.* 266:221–228.

Pradhan, S., Roy, S. N. & Pradhan, S. N. (1978) Correlation of behavioral and neurochemical effects of acute administration of cocaine in rats. *Life. Sci.* 22:1737–1744.

Pradhan, S. N. (1974) Aggression and central neurotransmistters. *Ann. Rev. Psychol.* 18:213–262.

Pycock, C. J., Donaldson, I. M. & Marsden, C. D. (1975) Circling behavior produced by unilateral lesions in the region of the locus coeruleus in rats. *Brain Res.* 97:317–329.

Rackham, A. & Wise, R. A. (1979) Independence of cocaine sensitization and amygdaloid kindling in the rat. *Physiol. Behav.* 22:631–633.

Rebec, G. V., Centore, J. M., White, L. K. & Alloway, K. D. (1985) Ascorbic acid and the behavioral response to haloperidol: Implications for the action of antipsychotic drugs. *Science* 227:438–441.

Reith, M. E., Allen, D. L., Sershen, H. & Lajtha, A. (1984) Similarities and differences between high-affinity binding sites for cocaine and imipramine in mouse cerebral cortex. *J. Neurochem.* 43:249–255.

Reith, M. E., Sershen, H., Allen, D. L. & Lajtha, A. (1983) A portion of [^{3}H]cocaine binding in brain is associated with serotonergic neurons. *Mol. Pharmacol.* 23:600–606.

Ritchie, J. M. & Greene, N. M. (1985) Local anesthetics. In: Gilman, A. G., Goodman, L. S., Rall, T. W. & Murad, F. (Eds.), *The pharmacological basis of therapeutics* (7th ed.). New York: Macmillan, 309–310.

Ritz, M. C. & Kuhar, M. J. (1989) Relationship between self-administration of amphetamine and monoamine receptors in brain: Comparison with cocaine. *J. Pharmacol. Exp. Ther.* 248: 1010–1017.

Ritz, M. C., Lamb, R. J., Goldberg, S. R. & Kuhar, M. J. (1987) Cocaine receptors on dopamine transporters are related to self-administration of cocaine. *Science* 237:1219–1223.

Roberts, D.C.S., Corcoran, M. E. & Fibiger, H. C. (1977) On the role of ascending catecholaminergic systems in intravenous self-administration of cocaine. *Pharmacol. Biochem. Behav.* 6:615–620.

Robinson, S. E. (1986) 6-hydroxydopamine lesion of the ventral noradrenergic bundle blocks the effect of amphetamine on hippocampal acetylcholine. *Brain Res.* 397:181–184.

Robinson, S. E. & Hambrecht, K. L. (1988) The effect of cocaine on hippocampal cholinergic and noradrenergic metabolism. *Brain Res.* 457:383–385.

Ross, S. B. & Renyi, A. L. (1967) Inhibition of the uptake of tritiated catecholamines by antidepressant and related agents. *Eur. J. Pharmacol.* 2:181–186.

Ross, S. B. & Renyi, A. L. (1969) Inhibition of uptake of 5-hydroxytryptamine in brain tissue. *Eur. J. Pharmacol.* 7:270–277.

Russell, R. D. & Stripling, J. S. (1985) Monoaminergic and local anesthetic components of cocaine's effects on kindled seizure expression. *Pharmacol. Biochem. Behav.* 22:427–434.

Ryan, L. J., Marton, M. E., Linder, J. C. & Groves, P. M. (1988) Cocaine, in contrast to d-amphetamine, does not cause axonal terminal degeneration in neostriatum and agranular frontal cortex of Long-Evans rats. *Life Sci.* 43: 1403–1409.

Sayers, A. C. & Handley, S. L. (1973) A study of the role of catecholamines in the response to various central stimulants. *Eur. J. Pharmacol.* 23:47.

Scheel-Kruger, J., Braestrup, C., Nielsen, M., Golembioska, K. & Mogilnicka, E. (1977) Cocaine: Discussion on the role of dopamine in the biochemical mechanism of action. In:

Ellinwood, E. H. & Kilbey, M. M. (Eds.), *Cocaine and other stimulants*. New York: Plenum Press, 373–407.

Schubert, J., Fyro, B., Nyback, H. & Sedvall, G. (1970) Effects of cocaine and amphetamine on the metabolism of tryptophan and 5-hydroxytryptamine in mouse brain in vivo. *J. Pharm. Pharmacol.* 22:860–877.

Scott, J. A. & Crews, F. T. (1985) Increase in serotonin-1 receptor density in rat cerebral cortex slices by stimulation of beta-adrenergic receptors. *Biochem Pharmacol.* 34:1585–1588.

Seiden, L. S. & Vosmer, G. (1984) Formation of 6-hydroxydopamine in caudate nucleus of the rat brain after a single large dose of methylamphetamine. *Pharmacol. Biochem. Behav.* 21: 29–31.

Sershen, H., Reith, M. E., Hashim, A. & Lajtha, A. (1984) Reduction of dopamine uptake and cocaine binding in mouse striatum by N-methyl-4-phenyl-1,2,3,6-tetrahydropyridine. *Eur. J. Pharmacol.* 102:175–178.

Sershen, H., Reith, M.E.A. & Lajtha, A. (1980) The pharmacological relevance of the cocaine binding site in mouse brain. *Neuropharmacology* 19: 1145–1148.

Slotkin, T. A., Salvaggio, M., Lau, C. & Kirksey, D. F. (1978) ^{3}H-dopamine uptake by synaptic storage vesicles of rat whole brain and brain regions. *Life Sci.* 22:823–830.

Stamford, J. A., Kruk, Z. L. & Millar, J. (1988) Stimulated limbic and striatal release measured by fast cyclic voltammetry: Anatomical, electrochemical and pharmacological characterization. *Brain Res.* 454:282–288.

Stockmeier, C. A., Martino, A. M. & Kellar, K. J. (1985) A strong influence of serotonin axons on beta-adrenergic receptors in rat brain. *Science* 230:323–325.

Stoof, J. C. & Kebabian, J. W. (1984) Two dopamine receptors: Biochemistry, physiology and pharmacology. *Life Sci.* 35:2281–2296.

Stripling, J. S. (1982) Origin of cocaine- and lidocaine-induced spindle activity within the olfactory forebrain of the rat. *Electroenceph. Clin. Neurophysiol.* 53:208–219.

Stripling, J. S. (1983) Cocaine and "pharmacologic kindling" in the rat. *Exp. Neurol.* 82:499–503.

Stripling, J. S. & Ellinwood, E. H., Jr. (1976) Cocaine: Physiological and behavioral effects of acute and chronic administration. In: Mulé, S. J. (Ed.), *Cocaine: Chemical, biological, clinical, social, and treatment aspects*. Cleveland: CRC Press, 167–185.

Stripling, J. S. & Hendricks, C. (1982) Effect of cocaine and lidocaine on the expression of kindled seizures in the rat. *Pharmacol. Biochem. Behav.* 16: 855–857.

Stripling, J. S. & Russel, R. D. (1985) Effect of cocaine and penylenetetrazole on cortical kindling. *Pharmacol. Biochem. Behav.* 23:573–581.

Swann, A. C., Heninger, G. R., Roth, R. H. & Maas, J. W. (1981) Differential effects of short and long term lithium on tryptophan uptake and serotonergic function in cat brain. *Life Sci.* 28:347–354.

Swann, A. C., Koslow, S. H., Katz, M. M., Maas, J. W., Javaid, J., Secunda, S. K. & Robins, E. (1987) Lithium carbonate treatment of mania. Cerebrospinal fluid and urinary monoamine metabolites and treatment outcome. *Arch. Gen. Psychiat.* 44:345–354.

Swerdlow, N. R., Vaccarino, F. J., Amalric, M. & Koob, G. F. (1986) The neural substrates for the motor-activating properties of psychostimulants: A review of recent findings. *Pharmacol. Biochem. Behav.* 25:233–248.

Tassin, J. P., Studler, J. M., Herve, D., Blanc, G. & Glowinski, J. (1986) Contribution of noradrenergic neurons to the regulation of dopaminergic (D₁) receptor denervation supersensitivity in the rat prefrontal cortex. *J. Neurochem.* 46:243–248.

Taylor, D. L., Ho, B. T. & Fagan, J. D. (1979) Increased dopamine receptor binding in rat brain by repeated cocaine injections. *Commun. Psychopharmacol.* 3:137–142.

Tennant, F. S. (1985) Effect of cocaine dependence on plasma phenylalanine and tyrosine levels and on urinary MHPG excretion. *Am. J. Psychiat.* 142:1200–1201.

Thierry, A. M., Tassin, J. P., Blanc, G. & Glowinski, J. (1976) Selective activation of the mesocortical DA system by stress. *Nature* 263:242–244.

Vrijmoed-de Vries, M. C. & Cools, A. R. (1985) Further evidence for the role of the caudate nucleus in programming motor and nonmotor behavior in Java monkeys. *Exp. Neurol.* 87:58–75.

Warren, P. F., Peat, M. A. & Gibb, J. W. (1984) The effects of a single dose of amphetamine and iprindole on the serotonergic system of the rat brain. *Neuropharmacology* 23: 803–806.

Weekley, L. B., Phan, T.-H., Narasimhachari, N., Johannessen, J. & Boadle-Biber, M. C. (1985) Effect of clonidine on the activity of tryptophan hydroxylase from rat brainstem following in vivo or in vitro treatment. *Biochem. Pharmacol.* 34:1549–1557.

Wetzel, G. T. & Brown, J. H. (1985) Presynaptic modulation of acetylcholine release from cardiac para-sympathetic neurons. *Am. J. Physiol.* 248:H33–H39.

Wilson, C. J., Juraska, J. M. & Groves, P. M. (1977) Alteration of the neuronal response to amphetamine in the neostriatum by pretreatment with a centrally acting anticholinergic. *Neuropharmacology* 16:455–461.

Wilson, M. C. & Schuster, C. R. (1973) Cholinergic influence on intravenous cocaine self-administration in rhesus monkey. *Pharmacol. Biochem. Behav.* 1:643–649.

Wise, R. A. (1980) Action of drugs of abuse on brain reward systems. *Pharmacol. Biochem. Behav.* 13(Supp. 1): 213–223.

Woolverton, W. L. & Balster, R. L. (1979) Reinforcement properties of some local anesthetics in rhesus monkeys. *Pharmacol. Biochem. Behav.* 11:669–672.

Woolverton, W. L. & Goldberg, L. E. (1984) The effects of selective dopamine (DA) receptor antagonists on the self-administration of cocaine and peribedil. *Fed. Proc.* 43:1036.

Woolverton, W. L. & Kleven, M. S. (1988) Multiple dopamine receptors and the behavioral effects of cocaine. In: Clouet, D., Ashgar, K. & Brown, R. (Eds.), *Mechanisms of cocaine abuse and toxicity.* NIDA Research Monograph 88, DHHS pub. no. 88-1585. Washington, D.C.: U.S. Government Printing Office, 160–184.

Woolverton, W. L. & Virus, R. M. (1989) The effects of D1 and D2 dopamine antagonist on behavior maintained by cocaine or food. *Pharmacol. Biochem. Behav.* 32:691–697.

Wong, D. T., Bymaster, F. P., Reid, L. R., Fuller, R. W., Perry, K. W. & Kornfeld, E. C. (1983) Effect of a stereospecific D2-dopamine agonist on acetylcholine concentration in corpus striatum of rat brain. *J. Neural Tran.* 58:55–67.

Yabase, M., Chinn, C., Charino, M. A. & Horita, A. (1989) Cocaine produces a cholinergically mediated analeptic and EEG arousal response in rabbits and rats. *Proc. West. Pharmacol. Soc.* 32:333.

Yasuda, R. P., Zahniser, N. R. &

Dunwiddie, T. V. (1984) Electrophysiological effects of cocaine in the rat hippocampus in vitro. *Neurosci. Lett.* 45:199–204.

Zito, K. A., Vickers, G. & Roberts, D.C.S. (1985) Disruption of cocaine and heroine self-administration following kainic acid lesions of the nucleus accumbens. *Pharmacol. Biochem. Behav.* 23: 1029–1036.

5

Imaging Techniques in the Investigation of the Effects of Cocaine in the Brain

Nora D. Volkow

Despite increasing awareness of the toxic and addicting properties of cocaine (Adams & Durrell, 1984; Cregler & Mark, 1986), there has been no systematic study of the mechanisms underlying the reinforcing and pathological actions of cocaine in the human brain. Multiple variables probably determine the detrimental effects of cocaine, from changes in life-style to direct actions of the drug in the brain (Fischman, 1984). Clinical experience with the effects of cocaine in other tissues suggests that some of the toxic properties of cocaine in the brain may be due to its actions on cerebral vessels (Volkow et al., 1988b). Indeed, there are several reports of cases in which cocaine ingestion has been associated with cerebrovascular accidents such as hemorrhages and infarcts (Brust & Richter, 1977; Cregler & Mark, in press; Langston & Langston, 1986; Lichtenfeld et al., 1984; Schwartz & Cohen, 1984; Tuchman et al., 1987). However, the profound neurochemical changes in the brain reported after single or repeated doses of cocaine are also probably implicated in some of the toxic actions of cocaine in addition to its reinforcing properties.

Until recently, direct interpretation of neurochemical findings with respect to the toxic and addictive properties of cocaine has been limited by differences between animals and humans and between in vitro and in vivo methods. Evaluation of neurochemical parameters in vivo in human beings has been limited to assessment of indirect measurements because of the inaccessibility of the brain. The recent development of imaging techniques, however, can now provide in vivo quantitative information about neurochemical and functional characteristics of the human brain. Advancement in imaging technology has made it feasible to quantify and locate neurochemical events to specific structures in the human brain. In this chapter, we will describe the basic principles of the main imaging modalities and their use in the investigation of the effects of cocaine and other drugs of abuse on the brain. We will relate these findings to those obtained using parallel strategies in animal studies.

Over the past few years, multiple techniques have evolved that allow noninvasive imaging of the living brain. These techniques can be divided into two categories: those that assess anatomical parameters of the brain and those that evaluate its functional and biochemical characteristics. The former category includes computerized axial tomography (CT scan) and nuclear magnetic resonance imaging instruments (NMR). Functional brain-imaging techniques include computerized electroencephalography (cEEG), single photon emission computed tomography (SPECT), and positron emission tomography (PET). The measurements obtained by these techniques represent different biological parameters that are quantified and located throughout the brain. Through the use of computers, these measurements can be transformed into images, which reveal different biological information depending on the technique used. These images can be obtained directly by measuring activity within the brain, such as in the axial techniques represented by CT scan, PET, SPECT, and NMR, or they can be obtained by monitoring the surface activity in the brain, as exemplified by the EEG.

COMPUTERIZED AXIAL TOMOGRAPHY

The CT scan provides axial images of regional anatomy of the brain. The images are obtained by applying an external radiation source. Radioactive rays are attenuated as they pass through the different tissues of the brain; the degree of attenuation depends on the density of the tissues. External detectors quantify the amount of radioactivity left (attenuation coefficients), and a computer reconstructs the images based on these coefficients (Ter Pogossian, 1977). These images have been useful in demonstrating brain pathology when structural damage has occurred as a result of stroke, hemorrhage, tumor, hydrocephalus, or dementia. Investigation of brain abnormalities in patients with histories of multiple drug abuse using CT scan has documented the occurrence of structural brain damage. The most common finding has been cortical atrophy. The structural changes seen in some of these patients have been interpreted as reflecting hemorrhages and infarcts associated with the abuse of drugs. These findings are difficult to interpret, however, because they occur in a small percentage of the population and because cortical atrophy is nonspecific. Furthermore, the structural damage could represent secondary, rather than direct, effects from the drugs, such as allergic reactions to contaminant material or emboli secondary to injection of small particles (Leeds et al., 1983).

In attempting to investigate toxic effects of cocaine in the brain, CT scans have been useful in demonstrating morphological changes in patients who developed neurological symptoms after cocaine consumption. In these cases the neurological symptoms appear to be the result of vascular pathology. Cocaine consumption has been associated with subarachnoid hemorrhages due to rupture of aneurysms (Lichtenfeld et al., 1984; Schwartz & Cohen, 1984), intracerebral hemorrhages (Caplan et al., 1982; Lowenstein et al., 1987; Nolte & Gelman, 1989; Tuchman et al., 1987; Wojak & Flamm, 1987), and cerebral infarction (Brust & Richter, 1977; Golbe & Merkin, 1986; Levine et al., 1987; Moen et al., 1987; Rowley et al., 1989; Weingarten, 1988). A case has also been reported of a newborn baby who developed a brain infarction within 24 hours of birth to a mother who had taken 1 gram of cocaine 15 hours before delivery (Chasnoff et al., 1986).

Though CT scans revealed brain pathology associated with cocaine in some cases, they have failed to show abnormalities where angiographic studies revealed vascular pathology (Altes-Capella et al., 1987). Failure to demonstrate abnormalities on CT scan with positive angiographic findings occurs mainly when patients are studied shortly after the vascular accident. The poor sensitivity of the CT scan to the early changes of a vascular accident should alert the clinician to the possibility of false negative findings with CT scan in patients with acute onset of neurologic symptoms after abuse of cocaine.

MAGNETIC RESONANCE IMAGING

Magnetic resonance imaging instruments (MRI) allow axial imaging of the brain without the use of ionizing radiation and with a better spatial resolution between gray and white matter structures than can be obtained with the CT scan. The method used for obtaining an image from the MRI is based on the magnetic properties of nucleons. Nucleons rotate about their axes in a random direction and, if placed in a static magnetic field, will orient into the field's line of induction. If tipped away from the vertical axis, these spinning nuclei will rotate (precession). In order to keep the spin, an external, electromagnetic radiation that matches the natural precessional frequency of the nuclei must be applied. By choosing relevant magnetic frequency, one can select specific nuclei, since each nucleus has a distinctive magnetic resonance frequency. The MRI instrument detects the energy liberated when the protons relax into their original state. The strength of the signal depends on the proton density of the section being examined. The time required for the proton to return to equilibrium is also measured by NMR and provides information on the magnetic characteristics of the surrounding tissue. Short relaxation time exists when water is closely bound to protein whereas slow relaxation time is seen when it is in the fluid state. Most of the medical NMR images have been obtained with resonances from hydrogen nuclei. By measuring the distribution of hydrogen, predominantly in water and fat, the different tissues can be imaged in a manner similar to that of a CT scan, yet with a much better resolution for white and gray matter: Gray matter contains 15% more water than white, whereas for a CT scan the difference in specific gravity between gray and white matter is only 0.2% (Brownell et al., 1982; Smith, 1983). In the future, with the development of high-field instruments, it may be feasible to obtain functional information with MRI; an image of phosphorus within the brain, for example, might reveal information about cellular energy stores.

There has not been any systematic study evaluating the effects of drugs of abuse with MRI. Isolated case reports of multiple drug abusers suggest that certain drugs like heroin, cocaine, and amphetamines can induce demyelinating lesions in the brain suggestive of vascular pathology in white matter tissue (Gawin et al., personal communication; Volkow et al., 1989b; Weingarten, 1988). The higher sensitivity of MRI over CT in detecting brain pathology makes it a better technique for locating structural changes associated with drug abuse.

COMPUTERIZED ELECTROENCEPHALOGRAPHY

The release of a neurotransmitter into the synapse and its binding to the receptor generates an electrical signal that is transmitted into the neuron. These electrical signals can be recorded, and their measurement generates the electroencephalographic signal. Electroencephalographic signals can be translated by computer into images that represent the electrical activity of various regions in the brain. The EEG is recorded from electrodes placed over the surface of the head. This limits the spatial resolution of the technique since precise localization of the electrical events is not feasible because what is recorded reflects an average of the electrical processes underlying the area recorded (Duffy et al., 1979).

Electrophysiological techniques have been very useful in investigating the effects of psychotropic drugs in the central nervous system. Several electrophysiological approaches have been used to investigate the effects of cocaine in the brain. Acute cocaine administration has been shown to produce prominent alterations, such as spindles, in limbic structures after discharges and seizures activity (Eidelberg et al., 1963). Cocaine has also been shown to desynchronize the electroencephalogram and to increase multiple unit activity in the brain stem reticular formation (Wallach & Gershon, 1971). Repeated administration of cocaine has been demonstrated to increase the electrophysiological responses recorded in several limbic structures favoring the occurrence of seizures at doses which had previously not produced them (Post & Kopanda, 1975). This phenomenon was described as analogous to the one of neurophysiological kindling. This "kindling phenomenon" appears to be related to the anesthetic properties of cocaine since similar electrophysiological findings have been reported with lidocaine (Wagman et al., 1968).

The assessment of the actions of cocaine on monoamine neuronal systems has profited from both extracellular and intracellular single-unit electrophysiological recording techniques (Lakoski & Cunningham, 1988). Studies in animals have focused on the investigation of the effects of acute administration of different doses of cocaine on the firing rate of monamine-containing neurons and their terminal projections throughout the brain. These studies have shown that intravenous administration of 0.06 to 4 mg/kg cocaine to rats produces an inhibition of the firing of neurons from the locus coeruleus, dorsal raphe nucleus, and ventral tegmental areas (Pitts & Marwah, 1988). The above centers, which contain high concentrations of norepinephrine, serotonin, and dopamine neurons, respectively, are particularly sensitive to the effects of cocaine and are also inhibited by acute administration of amphetamine. Though the chronic effects of cocaine on the firing rate of these centers have not been investigated there have been several reports documenting the effects of chronic or subchronic doses of amphetamine. Chronic amphetamine has been reported to increase the dose of amphetamine required to produce an inhibition of dopaminergic neurons in the ventral tegmental area and to reduce the inhibition of dopaminergic neurons when administering apomorphine, or dopamine (Pitts & Marwah, 1988). These effects could represent changes in dopaminergic receptors such as downregulation of dopamine autoreceptors due to chronic stimulation by amphetamine. The down regulation of the autoreceptors appears to be a temporary response dependent on the time since the last amphetamine administration. The similarity between cocaine and amphetamine with respect to the acute effects on monoaminergic neurons gives us reason to believe that similar regulatory mechanisms may occur with chronic administration of cocaine. In fact, studies using autoradiographic techniques directly to label the dopamine receptors have shown changes in presynaptic and postsynaptic dopamine receptors secondary to chronic cocaine administration.

Electrophysiological techniques have also been used to investigate the acute and chronic effects of cocaine administration in brain function (Phillips et al., 1975). A study of the effects of cocaine on the electroencephalographic signal in monkeys showed that acute administration of cocaine produced bidirectional changes in the EEG, with an initial decrease in EEG frequency occurring within the first 10 minutes followed by an increase in frequency 30–40 minutes after cocaine injection (Altschuler & Burch, 1976). To evaluate the effects of chronic cocaine on the EEG, Altschuler and Burch administered cocaine to these animals for eight months. Chronic treatment led to progressive decreases in EEG frequency during the 200 days of cocaine administration. It also led to changes in the response to acute cocaine administration with an accentuation of the initial decrease in EEG frequency occurring during the first 10 minutes post injection and a reduction in the increase in the EEG frequency occurring 30–40 minutes post cocaine injection. The slowing observed in the EEG frequency with chronic cocaine was interpreted as a pathological change, possibly related to the drug's cerebrovascular actions (Altschuler & Burch, 1976).

In contrast to research using animals, there have been very few systematic studies of brain electrophysiological changes in human chronic cocaine abusers. Electroencephalographic studies done in humans to investigate the effects of acute administration on EEG have reported an increase in beta frequency, particularly in frontal and temporal electrodes (Sano et al., 1988), that has been linked to the euphorigenic actions of cocaine.

SINGLE PHOTON EMISSION TOMOGRAPHY

The use of single photon emission computed tomography (SPECT) in conjunction with various radioactive compounds like iodine-123 labeled amphetamines or technetium-99 labeled hexamethylpropyl-eneamine oxime (HMPAO) has allowed axial measurements of CBF (cerebral blood flow) (Hill et al., 1984; Podreka et al., 1987). This is feasible because cerebral accumulation of these compounds is proportional to blood flow and they have a sufficient retention within the brain to allow for their measurement by the SPECT system. The measurements done with SPECT require the injection of a radioactive compound, which is measured within the organ of interest using multidetector systems that rotate around the subject or that are arranged in a ring-type device (Halama & Henkin, 1986). Though quantification or radioactivity and spatial resolution are not as precise as with positron emission tomography (PET), SPECT offers a less expensive alternative since no cyclotron is required to produce the radioactive tracers as with PET; radioactive tracers can be purchased from a pharmaceutical company. Until recently most of the work done with SPECT has been limited to assessment of cerebral blood flow, but there has been an increasing effort directed toward labeling compounds that can be used to monitor receptors in the brain (Eckelman et al., 1984; Kung et al., 1989; Weinberger et al., 1989).

Measurement of CBF using SPECT can be used to determine the effects of cocaine on cerebral circulation as well as to assess regional brain dysfunction. In the future when SPECT tracers for receptor imaging are validated, this technology could be used in the investigation of neurochemical changes occurring with chronic use of cocaine. Isolated case studies of the effects of chronic cocaine on cerebral blood flow done with SPECT have shown widespread defects in the accumulation of the radiotracers in the brain of cocaine abusers. These defects probably represent disruptions of cortical cerebral blood flow (O'Connel, personal communication).

POSITRON EMISSION TOMOGRAPHY (PET)

PET is a nuclear medicine instrument that incorporates principles of the autoradiographic and blood flow techniques (Volkow & Tancredi, 1986). It provides three-dimensional images of the brain with much better resolution than the EEG and SPECT. It is based on the intravenous injection of radioactive compounds that concentrate differentially within the brain in relation to the needs of the tissue for the particular substance injected. Several compounds can be injected, thus allowing the study of different biochemical and physiological variables, such as glucose metabolism, oxygen metabolism, CBF, protein synthesis, and neurotransmitters (Phelps et al., 1986; Volkow et al., 1988a). These compounds are labeled with radioactive isotopes that decay by liberating positrons. Once a positron is liberated, it travels for a short distance before losing its energy and colliding with an electron. The collision of the electron and the positron generates two gamma rays that travel in almost opposite directions. The positron camera is able to detect these two gamma rays and will count them only if they arrive simultaneously (coincidence time) in two detectors operating in coincidence. The emission of the two gamma rays that travel in opposite directions allows the location of the event within the volume covered by the two coincident detectors (Volkow et al., 1988a).

The isotopes most commonly used in PET are carbon-11 with a half-life of 20.4 minutes, oxygen-15 with a half-life of 2.03 minutes, fluorine-18 with a half-life of 110 minutes, and nitrogen-13 with a half-life of 9.96 minutes. The short half-lives of these compounds make their clinical use feasible. These isotopes can be used to label various radiopharmaceutical compounds that enable measurement of metabolism, neurotransmission, blood flow, and enzymes in the central nervous system. Most of the studies with PET have been done using an analog of glucose, deoxyglucose, labeled either with carbon-11 or fluorine-18. This compound, once trapped within the cell, remains there without being further metabolized, thus allowing the PET camera to detect the radioactivity in a steady-state condition. This measurement provides information on the rate of glucose metabolism by various brain areas (Bartlett et al., 1988; Reivich et al., 1985). Measurement of cerebral blood flow has also been accomplished using PET, most commonly by the use of oxygen-15 labeled water (Raichle et al., 1983; Fox et al., 1984). This is feasible because the concentration of oxygen-15 labeled water in the first seconds after injection reflects the blood flow of the area. Glucose metabolism and cerebral blood flow have been used as parameters of brain function, since the only source of energy in the brain is glucose and its delivery is dependent on cerebral blood flow (Siesjo, 1978). The existence of such a relationship has been documented in humans in whom increased regional blood flow of particular brain areas is elicited with mental (Risberg & Ingvar, 1973) and motor activities (Olsen, 1971). The flow-metabolic coupling has also been demonstrated at the neuronal level with rapid adjustment of flow to metabolic requirements (Silver, 1978).

Over the past few years, several compounds have been labeled with positron emitters and have been evaluated to monitor various neurotransmitters including dopamine, serotonin, and acetylcholine. Also, new methods have been developed to monitor enzyme concentration in the brain directly, as in the case of monoamine oxidase (Fowler et al., 1987). Though PET is a relatively new technique, it has already proven to be of value in detecting previously unrecognized abnormalities in patients with mental disorders (Volkow et al., 1988a; Volkow et al., 1985).

CEREBRAL BLOOD FLOW IN CHRONIC COCAINE USERS

The effects of chronic cocaine administration on cerebral blood flow was investigated using PET and oxygen-15-labeled water (Volkow et al., 1988a, 1988b). A group of 20 chronic cocaine abusers with a history of at least 6 months of continuous intravenous or freebase use was compared with a group of 24 normal controls. Patients were scanned initially when they first entered the hospital and again after 10 days off cocaine. This study revealed that chronic cocaine abusers had circumscribed areas of decreased blood flow located throughout the whole brain, but with a predominance in the anterior cortical areas and in the left hemisphere. These defects remained after 10 days of detoxification, suggesting that they were not related to withdrawal since by this time most of the withdrawal symptoms had subsided (Gawin & Kleber, 1984). The defects in cerebral blood flow were interpreted as representing circumscribed cerebrovascular accidents secondary to chronic cocaine abuse. Despite these widespread defects, the patients did not suffer from severe cognitive impairment or neurological symptoms. This discrepancy between the clinical symptomatology of the patients and their perfusion defects may have been due to a reserve in cerebral blood flow that allows decreases in perfusion without affecting brain functions.

Although this study systematically corroborates previous single case reports of strokes associated with cocaine, it still provides no clues to the mechanisms underlying the cerebrovascular effects seen in chronic cocaine abusers. Various explanation for these effects have been suggested, such as that (1) the sympathomimetic effects of cocaine induce direct vasoconstriction of cerebral vessels, leading to decreased cerebral blood flow, which, if severe, could produce ischemia and necrosis; (2) the sympathomimetic effects produce transient increases in blood pressure, which precipitate hemorrhagic episodes; (3) the defects in cerebral blood flow represent an allergic reaction to the drug or to its contaminants; or (4) the defects result from injection of small crystals in contaminated drugs, which could lead to embolic phenomena (Caplan et al., 1982; Chasnoff et al., 1986; Citron et al., 1970; Leeds et al., 1983; Rumbaugh et al., 1971). It is also important to keep in mind other variables that could produce some of these changes, such as combinations of cocaine with other drugs; the mixed use of alcohol and cocaine is common. This is particularly relevant since alcohol has been shown to induce vasoconstriction of cerebral blood vessels at levels that produce mild to moderate intoxication (Altura & Altura, 1983), and acute alcohol consumption has been associated with a higher incidence of strokes. (Altura & Altura, 1984; Gill et al., 1986; Hillborn & Kaste, 1981). The route of administration is also important, since both freebase and intravenous administration lead to the highest concentrations of drug in plasma (Jeffcoat et al., 1989; Jones, 1984). The high potency of the freebase "crack" may carry a particularly high risk for inducing cerebral vasospasm (Golbe & Merkin, 1986).

EFFECTS OF COCAINE ON ENERGY METABOLISM

The ability of cocaine to depress central nervous tissue activity has been well documented in vitro (Bollard & McIlwain, 1959). Several animal studies in vivo have also been conducted to assess the effects of acute cocaine administration on regional brain energy metabolism in vivo. One study of the effects of acute cocaine administration on global energy utilization by the brain showed that after 20 mg/kg of IV cocaine there was a decrease in the utilization of phosphate-rich compounds by the brain consistent with a 20% decrease in energy metabolism (Rogers & Nahorski, 1973). There was a concomitant increase in the concentration of glucose in the brain. Autoradiographic studies documenting regional differences in response to cocaine have reported conflicting results (London et al., 1986; Porrino et al., 1988; Trusk & Stein, 1988). However, there is a consensus that metabolic response of the brain to cocaine is dose related, and that there are regional differences in sensitivity to cocaine. Autoradiographic studies failed to replicate the decreases in metabolism reported based on phosphate utilization. In contrast, these studies have documented increases in glucose metabolism as well as increases in octanoate uptake, a marker for brain function (Rowley & Collins, 1985), in areas of the extrapyramidal system and in the prefrontal cortex. Some of these studies have also documented increases in metabolism in the nucleus accumbens (Porrino et al., 1988). That the latter regions are main components of the mesocortical limbic dopamine system confirms the high sensitivity of the dopaminergic system to acute cocaine administration.

The effects of acute cocaine administration in human subjects have been evaluated using PET and ^{18}F-deoxyglucose (FDG) in a group of chronic cocaine abusers who were given 40 mg of cocaine IV (London et al., 1988). This preliminary study reported a decrease in metabolism of FDG throughout the entire brain except in the cerebellum after cocaine administration. The results of the studies disagree with those of autoradiographic studies, which documented increases in glucose metabolism in well–localized areas. Similar discrepancies between rats and humans have been reported on the metabolic effects of acute pharmacological intervention for other dopaminergic agonists or antagonists such as amphetamine and haloperidol (Pizzolato et al., 1984; Volkow, et al., 1986; Wolkin et al., 1987). More studies are needed to assess whether the decreases in the metabolism secondary to acute cocaine administration represent blood flow changes or decreases in nervous tissue activity.

The effects of chronic cocaine use on human brain glucose metabolism have been investigated in a group of 10 subjects with a six-month history of either freebase or IV cocaine abuse. FDG was used to assess glucose metabolism, as well as [15]0-labeled water to assess cerebral blood flow (Volkow, 1988b; Volkow et al., 1988b). Only 4 of these subjects showed defects in the metabolic images similar to those observed with CBF images. The other 6 subjects showed relatively normal uptake for FDG despite abnormal CBF. Although they were not compared directly to a normative data set, these chronic cocaine abusers showed relative decreases in metabolism of the left frontal cortex. This decreased metabolism possibly relates to the marked degree of dysphoria experienced by these subjects, since lower metabolism of the left frontal cortex has been documented in depressed patients (Baxter et al., 1985). However, it could also represent a nonspecific effect (such as level of arousal) of the mental state of the subject while doing the procedure (Prohovnik et al., 1980).

EFFECTS OF COCAINE ON DOPAMINE RECEPTORS

Evidence from animal studies indicates that the reinforcing properties of cocaine are related to its effects on the dopamine system (Goeders & Smith, 1983) (for more detail, refer to the chapters by Swann and Wise). Similarly, addiction to cocaine is related to the effects of chronic cocaine on dopamine function (Dackis & Gold, 1985).

A large number of animal studies have investigated the effects of chronic cocaine abuse on the dopamine system. There is wide discrepancy among investigators' results (see reviews by Galloway, 1988, and Post et al., 1987). Some studies have shown that chronic cocaine administration leads to a persistent depletion of brain dopamine (DA) stores. For example, Trulson and Ulissey (1986) have reported that twice-daily administration of cocaine (10 mg/kg, IP [intraperitoneal]) for 10 days resulted in a significant decrease in DA, HVA, and DOPAC levels. These effects were observed for up to 60 days following termination of the chronic treatment. In contrast to these results, Kleven and Woolverton (1988) were unable to detect an effect of chronic cocaine administration on dopamine, serotonin, or major metabolities in the striatum, hippocampus, hypothalamus, or somatosensory cortex.

The data on the receptor effects of chronic cocaine administration are equally variable (see Post et al., 1987). Trulson and Ulissey (1986) found that [^{3}H]spiroperidol binding was significantly increased ($+24$ to $+36\%$) after chronic cocaine intoxication in animals tested 60 days after the last cocaine dose. In contrast, Dworkin et al. (1987) were unable to detect a change in postsynaptic receptor density (or affinity) 24 hours after cocaine termination in animals given cocaine (10 mg/kg IP) once daily for 8 or 14 days; however, these authors did observe a functional increase in D2 autoreceptor activity. Goeders and Kuhar (1987) showed that a similar regimen of cocaine over 15 days led to decreased sulpiride binding in the striatum when measured 24 hours after termination of cocaine administration. In studies done with d-amphetamine, a drug that shares many pharmacological actions with cocaine, chronic administration led to decreased binding of [^{3}H]spiroperidol (Hitzemann et al., 1980) 12 hours after amphetamine termination. In another study, chronic amphetamine was found to induce dopamine autoreceptor subsensitivity one day after drug discontinuation and supersensitivity one week after abstinence (Ellinwood & Lee, 1983).

In recent years emphasis has been placed on the development of dopamine agonists and antagonists for monitoring dopamine receptors in the human brain. In conjunction with PET, the most frequently used compound for the assessment of postsynaptic dopamine receptors has been ^{18}F-N-methylspiroperidol (^{18}FNMS) (Arnett et al., 1985). Binding of ^{18}FNMS by the brain has been shown to be selective for dopamine receptors after 40 min of injection, since at this time nonspecific binding of ^{18}FNMS and binding to serotonin receptors have washed out (Wong et al., 1987). This technique has demonstrated a decline of dopamine receptors with age (Wong et al., 1984) as well as varying degrees of receptor blockage by different concentrations of neuroleptics (Smith et al., 1988). Measurement of the uptake of ^{18}FNMS has proved useful in monitoring dopamine receptors within the brain, making it feasible to evaluate changes in dopamine receptors in human subjects who have been chronically exposed to cocaine.

We have conducted a preliminary study to assess the effects of chronic cocaine use on postsynaptic dopamine receptors using PET and ^{18}FNMS (Volkow et al., 1989a). Decreases in ^{18}FNMS uptake were revealed in chronic cocaine abusers tested within one week of last cocaine administration. We interpreted the decrease in ^{18}FNMS uptake as a reflection of decreases in dopamine receptors secondary to dopamine stimulation from cocaine. By inhibiting dopamine reuptake sites, cocaine induces transient increases in dopamine, which may lead to downregulation of the dopamine receptor. The same investigators report that after 4–6 weeks of cocaine withdrawal uptake of ^{18}NMSP returns to normal or to supernormal levels (Volkow et al., 1989a). These results indicate the dynamic nature of the changes in receptors induced by cocaine administration and withdrawal. In agreement with these findings is a preliminary PET study reporting decreased uptake of ^{18}F-dopa in two chronic cocaine abusers who were tested within one week of last cocaine consumption (Baxter et al., 1988).

These studies should be compared with studies of animals in which evaluation of the effects of chronic cocaine on dopamine receptors using radioactive-labeled antagonist has shown evidence of decreases in postsynaptic dopamine receptors 24 hours after termination of cocaine and of increases in postsynaptic dopamine receptors 60 days after termination of cocaine. In the future, studies evaluating the effects of acute versus chronic cocaine on dopamine receptors and their interactions with other transmitters may shed further light on the pharmacological actions of cocaine and on adaptive phenomena such as sensitization and tolerance.

COCAINE DISTRIBUTION IN THE BRAIN

Several studies have evaluated the binding characteristics of tritiated cocaine in the brains of animals. The results have shown that at least two types of receptors bind to cocaine: a high-affinity receptor that is sodium-sensitive and concentrates in dopamine-rich areas such as the striatum, and a lower-affinity receptor that appears to be located in cortical areas (Galloway, 1988).

With PET it is now feasible to label cocaine directly with a positron emitter and to monitor its binding and distribution in the brain of living organisms. A preliminary study was reported showing the distribution and binding characteristics of ^{11}C-cocaine in the brain of baboons (Fowler et al., 1988). This study reported a high uptake and clearance of cocaine from the brain with maximal peak of activity within 4–6 minutes of cocaine injection. Maximal concentration of the carbon-11 cocaine occurred in the basal ganglia. The binding of cocaine was prevented by preadministration of either cocaine or nomifensin. Since nomifensin is a norepinephrine and serotonin reuptake inhibitor, these studies suggest that cocaine binds predominantly to the dopamine reuptake sites. Binding was also observed in the heart during the first 10 minutes of the study. After 30 minutes there was almost no radioactivity in the brain or in the heart. In contrast, the liver and the bladder maintained relatively high levels of blood activity throughout the 90 minutes of the scan. Studies done in human subjects with ^{11}C-cocaine and PET have demonstrated binding characteristics similar to those seen in baboons (Fowler et al., 1989). Maximal binding of cocaine occurs within 4–8 minutes post injection, with rapid clearance of cocaine from the brain (less than 50% remaining after 20 minutes post injection). Cocaine bound predominantly to the basal ganglia where desipramine failed to inhibit its binding. The uptake and clearance of cocaine from the basal ganglia parallels the time sequence of the subjective euphoric response to the effects of cocaine (Cook et al., 1984). These results, though not conclusive, suggest that the euphoric response to cocaine in humans is mediated through cocaine binding to the dopamine reuptake site.

CONCLUSION

The new brain-imaging techniques have expanded our abilities to investigate the toxic effects of cocaine in the brain and the mechanisms underlying the reinforcing and addicting properties of cocaine. Although the cost of some of the techniques is very high (approximately $2,000 for a PET scan), they provide information that is not otherwise available, such as the measurement of regional brain function, evaluation of neurotransmitters and receptors, and assessment of pharmacokinetics within different brain areas in living human subjects. In the case of cocaine research, these techniques provide a way of establishing the link between the biological actions of cocaine in the brain and its behavioral effects such as euphoria and addiction.

ACKNOWLEDGMENT

Preparation of this chapter was supported by the U.S. Department of Energy under contract no. DE-AC02-76H000016.

REFERENCES

Adams, E. H. & Durell, J. (1984) Cocaine: A growing public health problem. In: Grabowski, J. (Ed.), Co- caine: Pharmacology, effects, and treatment of abuse. NIDA Research Monograph 50, DHHS pub. no. (ADM) 84-1326.

Washington, D.C.: Government Printing Office, 9–14.

Altes-Capella, J., Cabezudo-Artero, J. M. & Forteza-Rei, J. (1987) Complications of cocaine abuse. *Ann. Int. Med.* 107:940.

Altschuler H. L. & Burch, N. R. (1976) Cocaine dependence: Psychogenic and physiological substrates. In: Mule, S. J. (Ed.), *Cocaine: Chemical, biological, clinical, social and treatment aspects.* Cleveland: CRC Press, 135–147.

Altura, B. M. & Altura, B. T. (1983) Alcohol induced spasms of cerebral blood vessels: Relation to cerebrovascular accidents and sudden death. *Science* 220:331–333.

Altura, B. M. & Altura, B. T. (1984) Alcohol, the cerebral circulation and strokes. *Alcohol* 1:325–331.

Arnett, C. D., Fowler, J. S., Wolf, A. P., Shive, C. Y. & McPherson, D. W. (1985) ^{18}F-N-methylspiroperidol: The radioligand of choice for PET studies of the dopamine receptor in human brain. *Life Sci.* 36:2359.

Bartlett, E. J., Brodie, J. D., Wolf, A. P., Christman, D. R., Laska, E. & Meissner, M. (1988) Reproducibility of cerebral glucose metabolic measurements in resting human subjects. *J. Cereb. Blood Flow Metab.* 8:502–512.

Baxter, L. R., Phelps, M., Mazziotta, J. C., Schwartz, J. M., Gerner, R. H., Selin, C. E. & Sumida, R. M. (1985) Cerebral metabolic rate for mood disorders. *Arch. Gen. Psychiat.* 42:441–447.

Baxter, L. R., Schwartz, J. M., Phelps, M., Mazziotta, J. C., Barrio, J., Raucson, R., et al. (1988) Localization of neurochemical effects of cocaine and other stimulants in the human brain. *J. Clin. Psychiat.* 49:23–26.

Bollard, B. M. & McIlwain, H. (1959) Cocaine and procaine on the electrically stimulated metabolism of cerebral tissues. *Biochem. Pharmacol.* 2: 81–82.

Brownell, G., Budinger, T., Lauterbur, P. & Geer, P. (1982) Positron tomography and nuclear magnetic resonance imaging. *Science* 215:619–626.

Brust, J. D. & Richter, R. W. (1977) Stroke associated with cocaine abuse. *NY State J. Med.* 77:1473–1475.

Caplan, L. R., Hier, D. B. & Banks, G. (1982) Current concepts of cerebrovascular disease—stroke: Stroke and drug abuse. *Stoke* 13:869–872.

Chasnoff, I. J., Bussey, M. E., Savich, R. & Stack, C. M. (1986) Perinatal cerebral infarction and maternal cocaine use. *J. Pediatr.* 108:456–459.

Citron, B. P., Halpern, M., McCaron, M., Lundberg, G., McCormick, R., Pincus, I. J. et al. (1970) Necrotizing angiitis associated with drug abuse. *N. Engl. J. Med.* 283:1003–1011.

Cook, C. E., Jeffcoat, R. A. & Perez-Reyes, M. (1984) Pharmacokinetic studies of cocaine and phencyclidine in man. In: Barnett, G. & Chiang, N. C. (Eds.), *Pharmacokinetics and pharmacodynamics of psychoactive drugs.* Foster City, Calif.: Biomedical Publications, 48–74.

Cregler, L. L., & Mark, H. (1986) Medical complications of cocaine abuse. *N. Engl. J. Med.* 315:1495–1500.

Cregler, L. L. & Mark, H. (in press) Relations of stroke to cocaine abuse. *NY State J. Med.*

Dackis, C. A. & Gold, M. (1985) New concepts in cocaine addiction: The dopamine depletion hypothesis. *Neurosci. Biobehav. Rev.* 9:464–477.

Duffy, F. H., Burchfield, J. L. & Lombroso, C. T. (1979) Brain electrical activity mapping: A method for extending the clinical utility of EEG and EP data. *Ann. Neurol.* 5:309–332.

Dworkin, L. P., Peris, J., Yasuda, R. P. et al. (1987) Repeated cocaine administration results in supersensitivity of striatal D-2 dopamine autoreceptors to pergolide. *Life Sci.* 42:255–262.

Eckelman, W. C., Reba, R. C., Rzeszotarski, W. J. et al. (1984) External imaging of cerebral muscarinic acetyl choline receptors. *Science* 223: 291.

Eidelberg, E., Lesse, H. & Gault, F. P. (1963) An experimental model of temporal lobe epilepsy: Studies of the convulsant properties of cocaine. In: Glasser, G. H. (Ed.), *EEG and behavior.* New York: Basic Books, 272–283.

Ellinwood, E. H. & Lee, T. H. (1983) Effects of continuous systemic infusion of d-amphetamine on the sensitivity of nigral dopamine cells to apomorphine inhibition of firing rates. *Brain Res.* 272:379–383.

Fischman, M. (1984) The behavioral pharmacology of cocaine in humans. In: Grabowski, J. (Ed.), *Cocaine: Pharmacology, effects, and treatment of abuse.* NIDA Research Monograph 50, DHHS pub. no. (ADM) 84-1326. Washington, D.C.: Government Printing Office, 72–91.

Fowler, J. S., Macgregor, R. R., Wolf, A. P., Arnett, C. D., Dewey, S. L., Schlyer, D., et al. (1987) Mapping human brain monoamine oxidase A and B with C-suicide inactivators and positron emission tomography. *Science* 235:481–485.

Fowler, J. S., Volkow, N. D., Wolf, A. P., Dewey, S. L., Schyler, D., MacGregor, R., et al. (1989) Mapping cocaine binding sites in human and baboon brain in vivo. *Synapse.* 4:371–377.

Fowler, J. S., Wolf, A. P., Dewey, S. L., McaGregor, R., Schlyer, D.,

Christman, D., et al. (1988) Subcortical binding of cocaine in living baboon brain using PET. *Soc. Neurosci.* 338:8.

Fox, P. T., Mintun, M. A., Raichle, M. E. & Herscovitch, P. (1984) A noninvasive approach to quantitative functional brain mapping with $H_2^{15}0$ and positron emission tomography. *J. Cereb. Blood Flow Metab.* 4:329–333.

Galloway, M. P. (1988) Neurochemical interaction of cocaine with dopaminergic systems. *TIPS* 9:451–454.

Gawin, F. H. & Kelber, H. D. (1984) Cocaine abuse treatment: Open pilot trial with desipramine and lithium carbonate. *Arch. Gen. Psychiat.* 41:903–910.

Gill, J. F., Zezulka, A. V., Shipley, M. J., Surinder, K., Gill, M. B. & Beevers, D. G. (1986) Stroke and alcohol consumption. *N. Engl. J. Med.* 313: 1044–1045.

Goeders, N. E. & Kuhar, M. J. (1987) Chronic cocaine induces opposite changes in dopamine receptors in the striatum and nucleus accumbens. *Alcohol Drug Res.* 7:207–216.

Goeders, N. E. & Smith, J. E. (1983) Cortical dopaminergic involvement in cocaine reinforcement. *Science* 221:773–775.

Golbe, L. I. & Merkin, M. D. (1986) Cerebral infarction in a user of freebase cocaine ("crack"). *Neurology* 36:1602–1604.

Halama, J. R. & Henkin, R. E. (1986) Single photon emission computed tomography (SPECT) In: Freeman, L. M. (Ed.), *Freeman and Johnson's clinical radionuclide imaging.* Orlando: Grune and Stratton, 1529–1654.

Hill, R. C., Magistretti, P. L. & Holman, B. L. (1984) Assessment of regional cerebral blood flow in stroke using SPECT and N-isopropyl-(I-123 iodoamphetamine (IMP). *Stroke* 15:40–45.

Hillborn, M. & Kaste, M. (1981) Ethanol intoxication a risk factor for ischemic brain infarction in adolescents and young adults. *Stroke* 12:422–425.

Hitzemann, R. J., Wu, J., Hom, D. & Loh, H. H. (1980) Brain locations controlling the behavioral effects of chronic amphetamine in intoxication. *Psychopharmacology* 72:93–101.

Jeffcoat, R. A., Perez-Reyes, M., Hill, J. M., et al. (1989) Cocaine dispostion in humans after intravenous injection, nasal insufflation (snorting) or smoking. *Drug. Metab. Disp.* 17:153–159.

Jones, R. T. (1984) The pharmacology of cocaine. In: Grabowski, J. (Ed.), *Cocaine: Pharmacology, effects, and treatment of abuse.* NIDA Research Monograph 50, DHHS pub. no. (ADM) 84-1326. Washington, D.C.: Government Printing Office, 34–52.

Kleven, M. S., Woolverton, W. C. & Seiden, L. S. (1988) Lack of long-term monoamine depletions following repeated or continuous exposure to cocaine. *Brain Res. Bull.* 21:233–237.

Kung, H. F., Pan, S., Kung, M. P. et al. (1989) In vitro and in vivo evaluation of (^{123}I) IBZM: A potential CNS dopamine D-2 receptor imaging agent. *J. Nucl. Med.* 30:88–92.

Lakoski, J. M. & Cunningham, K. A. (1988) Cocaine interaction with central monaminergic systems: Electrophysiological approaches *TIPS* 9:177–180.

Langston, W. J. & Langston, E. B. (1986) Neurological consequences of drug abuse. In: Asburg, A. K., McKhann, G. M. & McDonald, W. I. (Eds.), *Diseases of the nervous system.* Philadelphia: W. B. Saunders, 1333–1340.

Leeds, N., Malhotra, V. & Zimmerman, R. (1983) The radiology of drug addiction affecting the brain. *Sem. Roentgenology* 18:227–233.

Levine, S. R., Washington, J. M., Jefferson, M. F., Kieran, S. N., Moen, M., Feit, H. & Welch, K.M.A. (1987) "Crack" cocaine-associated stroke. *Neurology* 37:1849–1853.

Lichtenfeld, P. J., Rubin, D. B., & Feldman, R. S. (1984) Subarachnoid hemorrhage precipitated by cocaine snorting. *Arch. Neurol.* 41:223–224.

London, E. D., Gascella, N. G., Wong, D. F., Sano, M., Dannals, R. F., Links, J. et al. (1988) Acute cocaine decreases regional cerebral glucose utilization in human substance abusers. *J. Nucl. Med.* 29:840.

London, E. D., Wilkerson, G., Goldberg, S. R. & Risner, M. E. (1986) Effects of L-cocaine on local cerebral glucose utilization in the rat. *Neurosci. Let.* 68:73–78.

Lowenstein, D. H., Massa, S. M., Rowbotham, M. C., Collins, S. D., McKinney, H. E., & Simon, R. P. (1987) Acute neurologic and psychiatric complications associated with cocaine abuse. *Am. J. Med.* 83:841–846.

Moen, M., Levine, S. R., Washington, J. M., Jefferson, M. F., Kieran, S. N., Moen, M., et al. (1987) "Crack" cocaine-associated stroke. *Neurology* 37(Suppl. 1):372.

Notle K. B., & Gelman, B. B. (1989) Intracerebral hemorrhage associated with cocaine abuse. *Arch. Pathol. Lab. Med.* 113:812–813.

Olsen, J. (1971) Contralateral focal increase of cerebral blood flow in man during arm work. *Brain* 94:635–646.

Phelps, M. E., Mazziotta, J. C. & Schelbert, H. (1986) *Positron computed tomography.* New York: Raven Press.

Phillips, P. E., Altshuler, H. L.,

Sanders, D. W. & Burch, N. R. (1975) The effects of chronic cocaine hydrochloride administration on the primate electroencephalogram. *Pro. Soc. Neurosci.* 1:284.

Pitts, D. K. & Marwah, J. (1988) Cocaine and central monoaminergic neurotransmission. A review of electrophysiological studies and comparison to amphetamine and antidepressants. *Life Sci.* 42:949–968.

Pizzolato, G., Soncrant, T. T. & Rapoport, S. I. (1984) Haloperidol and cerebral metabolism in the conscious rat: Relation to pharmacokinetics. *J. Neurochem.* 43:724–732.

Podreka, I., Suess, E., Goldenber, G., Stein, M., Brucke, T., Muller, Ch., et al. (1987) Initial experience with technetium-99m HM-PAO brain SPECT. *J. Nucl. Med.* 28:1657–1666.

Porrino, L. J., Domer, F. R., Crane, A. M. & Sokoloff, L. (1988) Selective alterations in cerebral metabolism within the mesocortico limbic dopaminergic system produced by acute cocaine administration in rats. *Neuropsychopharmacology*, 1:109–118.

Post, R. M. & Kopanda, R. T. (1975) Cocaine, kindling and reverse tolerance. *Lancet* i:409.

Post, R. M., Weiss, S. R., Port, A. & Uhale, T. (1987) Chronic cocaine administration: Sensitization and kindling effects. In: Fischer, S. & Haskin, A. (Eds.), *Cocaine: Clinical and biobehavioral aspects*. New York: Oxford University Press, 109–173.

Prohovnik, I., Kakansson, K. & Risberg, J. (1980) Observations on the functional significance of regional cerebral blood flow in resting normal subjects. *Neuropsychologia* 18:203–217.

Raichle, M. E., Martin, W. R., Herscovitch, P., Minton, M. A. & Markham, J. (1983) Brain blood flow measured with intravenous $H_2^{15}O$. *J. Nucl. Med.* 24:790–798.

Reivich, M., Alavi, A., Wolf, A., Fowler, J., Russell, J., Arnett, C., et al. (1985) Glucose metabolic rate kinetic model parameter determination in man: The lumped constants and rate constants for ^{18}F-Fluorodeoxyglucose and ^{11}C-Deoxyglucose. *J. Cereb. Blood Flow Metab.* 5:179–192.

Risberg, J. & Ingvar, D. H. (1973) Patterns of activation in the gray matter of the dominant hemisphere during memorizing and reasoning. *Brain* 96: 737–756.

Rogers, K. J. & Nahorski, S. R. (1973) Depression of cerebral metabolism by stimulant doses of cocaine. *Brain Res.* 57:255–258.

Rowley, H. & Collins, R. C. (1985) ^{14}C Octanoate: A fast functional marker of brain activity. *Brain Res.* 335:326–329.

Rowley, H. A., Lowenstein, D. H., Rowbotham, M. C. & Simon, R. P. (1989) Thalamomesencephalic strokes after cocaine abuse. *Neurology* 39:428–430.

Rumbaugh, C. L., Bergeron, T., Fang, H. & McCormick, R. (1971) Cerebral angiographic changes in the drug abuse patient. *Radiology* 1010:335–344.

Sano, M., Cascella, N., Glover, B., Herning, R. & London, E. (1988) EEG and subjective responses to intravenous cocaine in human substance abusers. *Neuroscience* 388.16:963.

Schwartz, K. A. & Cohen, J. A. (1984) Subarachnoid hemorrhage precipitated by cocaine snorting. *Arch. Neurol.* 41:705.

Siesjo, B. K. (1978) *Brain energy metabolism*. New York: John Wiley & Sons.

Silver, I. A. (1978) Cellular microenvironment in relation to local blood flow. In: *Cerebral vascular smooth muscle and its control*. New York: Elsevier Excerpta Medica, North-Holland.

Smith, F. (1983) Nuclear magnetic resonance in the investigation of cerebral disorder. *J. Cereb. Blood Flow Metab.* 3:263–269.

Smith, M., Wolf, A. P., Brodie, J. D., et al. (1988) Serial [18]F N-methylspiroperidol PET studies to measure changes in antipsychotic drugs D2 receptor occupancy in schizophrenic patients. *Biol. Psychiat.* 23:653–663.

Ter Pogossian, M. (1977) Basic principles of computed axial tomography. *Sem. Nucl. Med.* 7:109–127.

Trulson, M. T. & Ulissey, M. J. (1986) Chronic cocaine administration decreases dopamine synthesis rate and increases ^{3}H spiroperidol binding in rat brain. *Brain Res. Bull.* 19:35–38.

Trusk, T. C. & Stein, E. (1988) Effects of heroin and cocaine on brain activity in rats using ^{14}C octanoate as a fast functional tracer. *Brain Res.* 438:61–66.

Tuchman, A. J., Daras, M., Salzal, P. & Mangiardi, J. (1987) Intracranial hemorrhage after cocaine abuse (letter). *JAMA* 257:1175.

Van Dyke, C. & Byck, R. (1982) Cocaine. *Sci. Am.* 246:128–141.

Volkow, N. D. (1988a) Effects of alcohol and cocaine on cerebral blood flow as measured with positron emission tomography. In: Takahashi, R., Flor Henry, P., Gruzelier, J. & Shinkhi, N. (Eds.), *Cerebral dynamics, laterality, and psychopathology*. Amsterdam: Elsevier.

Volkow, N. D. (1988b) Brain metabolism in chronic cocaine users. *Proceedings of the American Psychiatric Association Annual Meeting*, 117.

Volkow, N. D., Brodie, J. D., & Gomez-Mont, F. (1985) Application of positron emission tomography to psychiatry. In: Reivich, M. & Alavi, A. (Eds.), *Positron emission tomography*. New York: Alan R. Liss, 311–328.

Volkow, N. D., Brodie, J. D., Wolf, A. P. et al. (1986) Brain metabolism in predominantly never treated schizophrenics before and after acute neuroleptic. *J. Neuro. Neurosurg. Psych.* 49:1199–1202.

Volkow, N. D., Fowler, J., Wolf, A. P., Dewey, S., Schlyer, D., Logan, J., et al. (1989a) Effects of chronic cocaine on dopamine receptors. *J. Cereb. Blood Flow Metab.* 9:S 111.

Volkow, N. D., Mullani, N. & Bendriem, B. (1988a) PET intrumentation and clinical research. *Am. J. Physiol. Imaging* 3:142–153.

Volkow, N. D., Mullani, N., Gould, L., Adler, S. & Krajewski, K. (1988b) Cerebral blood flow in chronic cocaine users. *Br. J. Psychiat.* 152:641–648.

Volkow, N. D. & Tancredi, L. (1986) Positron emission tomography: Technological assessment. *Int. J. of Technology Assessment in Health Care* 2:577–594.

Volkow, N. D., Valentine, A. & Kulkarni, M. (1989b) Radiological and neurological changes in the drug abuse patient: A study with MRI. *J. Neuroradiol.* 15:288–293.

Wagman, I. H., De Jong, R. H., & Prince, D. A. (1968) Effects of lidocaine on spontaneous cortical and subcortical electrical activity. *Arch. Neuro.* 18:277–290.

Wallach, M. B. & Gershon, S. (1971) A neuropsychopharmacological comparison of d-amphetamine, L-dopa and cocaine. *Neuropharmacology* 10:743–752.

Weinberger, D. R., Gibson, R. E., Coppola, R., Jones, D. W., Braun, A.

R., Mann, U., et al. (1989) Disbribution of muscarinic receptors in patient with dementia: A controlled study of ^{123}I QNB and SPECT. *J. Cereb. Blood Flow Metab.* 9:5537.

Weingarten, K. (1988) Cerebral vasculitis associated with cocaine abuse or subarachnoid hemorrhage? *JAMA* 259: 1648–1649.

Wojack, J. C. & Flamm, E. S. (1987) Intracranial hemorrhage and cocaine use. *Stroke* 18:712–713.

Wolkin, A., Angrist, B., Wolf, A. P., Brodie, J., Jordan, B., Jaeger, J., et al. (1987) Effects of amphetamine on local cerebral metabolism in normal and schizophrenic subjects as determined by positron emission tomography. *Psychopharmacology* 92:241–246.

Wong, D. F., Giedde, A., Dannals, R., Lever, J., Ravert, H., Wilson, A. et al. (1987) Quantification of dopamine and serotonin receptors in living human brain. *J. Nucl. Med.* 28:611.

Wong, D. F., Wagner, H. N., Dannals, R., Links, J. M., Frost, J. J., Ravert, H. T., et al. (1984) Effects of age on dopamine and serotonin receptors measured by positron emission tomography in the living human brain. *Science* 226:1391–1396.

6

Pharmacology of Cocaine

Charles Ashley and Robert A. Hitzemann

Cocaine has local anesthetic effects and blocks monoamine reuptake. Although pharmacological studies have investigated both actions (Ritchie & Greene, 1980), inhibition of monoamine reuptake has been more specifically linked to cocaine's reinforcing and addicting effects.

In this chapter we will review these actions with respect to cocaine's ability to inhibit the dopamine reuptake site. We have chosen this approach because it is generally assumed that the brain's dopamine systems mediate the reinforcing properties of cocaine (Koob et al., 1987). Ritz et al. (1987) have shown that the cocaine receptors associated with self-administration of cocaine are the dopamine and not the serotonin or norepinephrine transporters. The cocaine K_i (affinity constant for the binding of the unlabeled ligand to the same site as the radioligand) for inhibition of the dopamine transporter was found to be 0.65 μM. Assuming that the inhibition of transport must be greater than 90% to facilitate reinforcement, the concentration of cocaine at the transporter site would have to be approximately 2.5 μM or 750 ng/ml. A conservative estimate of the brain:plasma ratio for cocaine is 5:1 (see Benuck et al., 1987); thus, to obtain a brain concentration of 750 ng/ml, a plasma concentration of 150 ng/ml is required. This concentration should be contrasted with the concentration of 10 mg/ml or 33 mM required to produce local anesthesia. In the following review, we will use 150 ng/ml as the benchmark concentration of cocaine and examine the relationships among different routes of administration, metabolism, and this benchmark concentration. To begin this inquiry, we will examine the structure of cocaine, its metabolites, and related alkaloids.

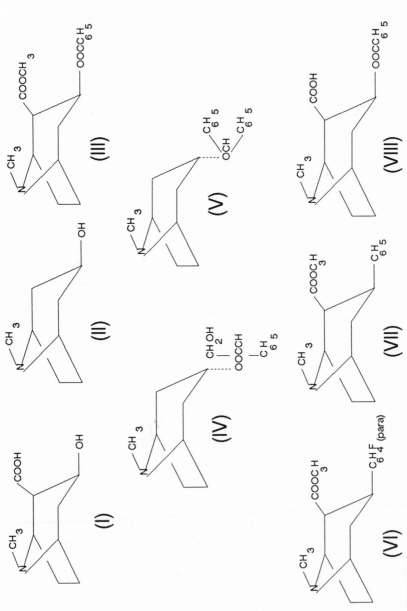

FIGURE 6.1

The structures of cocaine and related compounds.

(I) = ecgonine; (II) = tropine; (III) = cocaine; (IV) = atropine; (V) = benztropine; (VI) = WIN 35,065–2; (VII) = WIN 35,428; (VIII) = benzoylecgonine.

COCAINE STRUCTURE

Cocaine is the methyl ester benzoate derivative of the alkaloid ecgonine (I) which is structurally similar to tropine (II) (Figure 6.1). Thus, cocaine (III) has some structural similarity to atropine (IV) and the synthetic anticholinergic benztropine (V). Cocaine is optically active with the ($-$) isomer being more than 200 times more potent than the ($+$) isomer in inhibiting dopamine transport (Ritz et al., 1987). The similarity in structure between cocaine and benztropine is of interest in that both drugs are potent inhibitors of dopamine transport. The K_i for benztropine has been reported to be 120 nM (Horne et al., 1971). Cocaine, on the other hand, has little intrinsic anticholinergic activity and is a weak inhibitor of high affinity choline transport ($K_i = 250$ μM, Ritz et al., 1987). The benzoylester linkage is not required for cocaine-like activity. the cocaine analogs WIN 35,428 (VI) and WIN 35,065-2 (VII) are both more potent than cocaine as inhibitors of cocaine binding and dopamine transport (Reith et al., 1985). In man, the main metabolites of cocaine are ecgonine methyl ester, benzoylecgonine (VIII), and ecgonine (I). As reflected in the high brain:plasma ratio, cocaine is a hydrophobic molecule; the octanol/buffer partition coefficient over the range of 0.1 to 1 μg is 7.6 (Nayak et al., 1976).

ROUTES OF COCAINE ADMINISTRATION AND ABSORPTION

Though several factors probably contribute to the self-administration of cocaine, we will focus on cocaine's ability to block the dopamine transporter, since inhibition of dopamine transport appears to be a necessary condition for reinforcement. Within this context we will discuss the factors that are necessary to maintain a sufficient plasma concentration to inhibit dopamine transport. Figure 6.2 illustrates the dynamic interrelationships among absorption, distribution binding, metabolism, and excretion of a drug and the drug concentration at its site of action (which for our purposes will be the dopamine transporter).

Cocaine is generally administered orally, intranasally, intravenously, or by smoking. Figure 6.3 (adapted from Van Dyke &

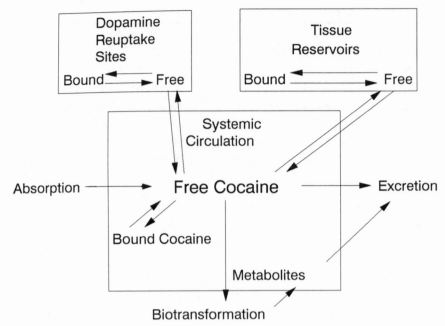

FIGURE 6.2
The pharmacokinetic relationships that determine the concentration of co-caine at its site of action, the dopamine transporter.

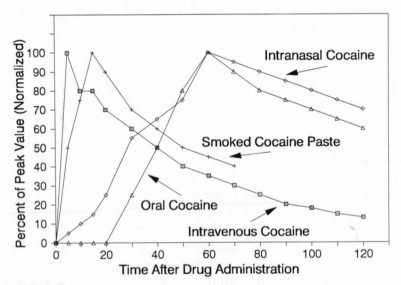

FIGURE 6.3
The rates of cocaine absorption from various routes of administration (adapted from Van Dyke and Byck, 1982).
The peak value refers to the peak plasma level, normalized to 100% for each route of administration.

Byck, 1982) illustrates the differences in the rate of absorption from each of these routes measured as the appearance of cocaine in the plasma. This type of graph was made possible by the development of a sensitive assay for cocaine (Jatlow & Bailey, 1975). Perhaps the most interesting aspect of this assay scheme was the rapid addition of fluoride to the sample to inhibit plasma pseudocholinesterase, which can rapidly metabolize cocaine. Van Dyke et al. (1978) compared intransasal versus oral administration of 2 mg/kg cocaine in four volunteers. For oral administration the cocaine was formulated as a gelatin capsule to prevent absorption from the oropharynx. For nasal administration, the cocaine was formulated as a 10% solution of cocaine hydrochloride, which was applied topically. After nasal administration, significant levels were detected at 15 minutes, and after oral administration, at 30 minutes. These time periods parallel the subjective feelings of "high" from the cocaine.

In both cases, the initial euphoric feelings were associated with plasma levels (36 ng/ml[nasal] and 54 ng/ml[oral]) that were significantly below the concentration thought to be necessary to insure inhibition of dopamine transport. From both routes of administration, the peak plasma level was reached at 1 hour and there was no significant difference between routes of administration in peak plasma level. The average peak levels obtained in this study (160 to 200 ng/ml) are close to or slightly above our benchmark concentration of 150 ng/ml. Javaid et al. (1978) administered cocaine intranasally by "snorting" a powder rather than by topically applying cocaine solution as in the Van Dyke et al. (1978) study. The peak plasma level of cocaine was reached at 30 minutes after administration of cocaine doses of 16, 64, and 96 mg; the peak levels obtained were 46, 115, and 206 ng/ml, respectively. Javaid et al. concluded that the difference in the time to maximum plasma concentration between their study and that of Van Dyke et al. (1978) may be due to the fact that since cocaine is a potent vasoconstrictor, slight differences in the mode of administration might markedly alter the rate of absorption. Jeffcoat et al (1989) also administered cocaine HCl intranasally ($N = 4$, 94 mg cocaine base) to healthy, recreational users. The peak plasma concentration (220 ng/ml) was obtained after 45 minutes and the elimination half-time was 78 minutes. Less than 1% was excreted unchanged in the urine. The estimated bioavailability by this route was 80 ± 13%.

The doses of cocaine administered in these studies are in general significantly greater than the usual single intranasal dose; such doses typically average 0.3 to 0.7 mg/kg (Siegel, 1984). However, even at these dose levels, one can rapidly build a plasma concentration of 150 ng/ml. If one assumes an administration of 1 dose/30 min, a fractional bioavailability of 30%, and a clearance of 33 ml/min/kg (Chow et al., 1985), then a dose of only 0.5 mg/kg would be sufficient to obtain a steady-state plasma concentration of 150 ng/ml after 4 to 5 doses. This relatively modest pattern of repeated drug use is consistent with the pattern of use found in the social-recreational user. The fractional bioavailability of cocaine may be dose-dependent. However, Javaid et al. (1983) noted that bioavailability increased on average in four subjects from 0.28 to 0.57 as the dose was increased from 64 to 96 mg. These authors argued that this phenomenon may simply reflect a greater amount of drug for absorption at the higher dose since the cocaine was administered as a 100 mg powder (cocaine plus lactose to 100 mg).

Administration of cocaine by intravenous (IV) injection or smoking delivers a cocaine bolus of high concentration to the brain, which results in an intense, highly pleasurable, but short-lived euphoric experience. Associated with this bolus of high concentration, the "nonspecific" effects of cocaine (e.g., local anesthetic effects) may contribute to this intense euphoric phenomenon. And, indeed, some local anesthetics devoid of transport inhibiting properties have been shown in animals to have reinforcing activity (Ford & Balster, 1977; Hammerbeck & Mitchell, 1978). Intravenous administration of 0.6 mg/kg of cocaine HCl over a period of 1 minute will produce peak plasma levels in the range of 300 to 400 ng/ml (Fischman & Schuster, 1982). Peak plasma concentration is reported to occur at 5 minutes post cocaine injection and it parallels the occurrence of the subjective response to cocaine (Javaid et al., 1978). Similarly, a recent study has also shown that IV administration of 23 mg of cocaine HCl in 3 ml saline over a 1 minute period produced a peak plasma concentration of 180 ng/ml approximately 5 minutes post injection (Jeffcoat et al., 1989). Bioavailability from this route (from the plasma perspective) is obviously 100% and thus more efficient than intranasal or oral administration. Assuming that clearance is not greatly affected by the route of administration (see the next section), then four to five doses of approximately 0.1 mg/kg IV/30 min would, in the average subject, be sufficient to insure inhibition of transport activity. Given that the IV abuse of cocaine is frequently associated with dosing levels at least an order of magnitude higher than 0.1 mg/kg, plasma levels of 150 ng/ml will be easily met during a "run" by most IV users.

The smoking of cocaine, especially freebase cocaine, is an efficient method of delivering a cocaine bolus of high concentration to the brain (Jeri et al., 1978; Paly et al., 1982; Siegel, 1984). As noted by Jones (1984), the alveoli of the lungs provide an enormous surface area for absorption of the volatilized cocaine. Freebase cocaine is much more stable than cocaine HCl during the pyrolization process, and thus the more desirable form for smoking (Jones, 1984). The time for delivery (to the brain) by smoking is approximately 8 sec as compared to a delivery time of 16 sec by IV injection into the arm. The great delivery time for IV injection is not only associated with a greater volume of distribution but also with a much greater likelihood of significant metabolism. Peak plasma concentration is reported to occur at 5 minutes post injection at which point the subject experiences the maximum "high" from the drug.

The doses of cocaine administered to small laboratory animals are generally much greater than their clinical equivalent. The differences in dose probably do not reflect any significant difference in absorption, but rather reflect the large differences in the volumes of distribution and the rates of metabolism. The differences in dose may, at first, seem startling. For example, in rats allowed daily access to cocaine (0.75 mg/kg, IV/injection) on a continuous reinforcement schedule, the total dose administered during a 3-hour trial was nearly 30 mg/kg (Koob et al., 1987). It is of interest to note that in this study the total dose administered was relatively constant over time for repeated daily doses and that if the dose/injection was doubled or halved, the rate of responding appropriately changed to maintain a constant total dose. Although the plasma and/or brain concentrations of cocaine were not measured in this study, we can certainly assume that the brain concentrations were in excess of that required to inhibit dopamine transport. This conclusion is consistent with the known pharmacokinetic data on the disposition of IV-administered cocaine in rodents. Extrapolating from the data of Nayak et al. (1976), it appears that a single IV dose of 0.75 mg/kg would result in a brain concentration of approximately 750 ng/g, 15 minutes after injection.

For the study of cocaine's effects on unconditioned behavior, the intraperitoneal (IP) route of administration is frequently used. Benuck et al. (1987) have recently examined the pharmacokinetics of IP-administered cocaine to mice. The mice were given 10 or 25 mg/ kg cocaine HCl. Peak brain levels for both the 10 and 25 mg/kg doses (2.6 and 6.7 μg/g, respectively) appeared within 5 minutes of injection. The average brain/plasma ratio was 7. At the time of peak brain cocaine concentrations, the brain levels of the major metabolite benzoylecgonine were 2% or less than those of cocaine. This is in marked contrast to the situation in plasma, where 5–10 minutes after injection the benzoylecgonine concentrations were higher than those of cocaine. Even at 1 hour after cocaine administration, at a time when the brain cocaine levels have dropped >90% from their peak levels, the brain concentration of benzoylecgonine is < than that of cocaine. Thus, the polar metabolite of cocaine, benzoylecgonine (structure VIII in Figure 6.1), has only limited uptake across the blood-brain barrier. This point is not entirely trivial considering that benzoylecgonine, which has local anesthetic activity, may contribute to the behavioral effects associated with high-dose cocaine abuse, although the preceding data suggest that this is unlikely providing that the blood-brain barrier remains intact. Overall, it should be noted that the IP route of administration promptly delivers cocaine to the brain; in the doses generally administered within the context of the laboratory experiment (10 to 30 mg/kg), the peak and peri-peak levels are sufficient to inhibit dopamine transport.

The subcutaneous (s.c.) route of administration is frequently used for animal drug studies, especially those requiring chronic administration. As might be expected, the peak plasma and brain levels after s.c. administration are significantly delayed (compared to IP administration), with peak levels being found at approximately 4 hours (Nayak et al., 1976). Most certainly this phenomenon reflects a prolonged course of absorption from the site of injection, due to cocaine's vasoconstrictor properties.

Our discussion of both clinical and animal studies has largely focused on single-dose experiments. From the perspective of cocaine abuse, however, it is the pharmacokinetics of chronic, intense cocaine administration that is of the most interest. Almost no clinical data are available because of the obvious difficulties in conducting a well-controlled clinical trial of repeated cocaine administration. Two recent reviews of cocaine pharmacology and patterns of abuse (Grabowski, 1984; Kozel & Adams, 1985) cite no studies of pharmacokinetics in the chronic abuser. Surprisingly, the situation regarding animal studies is only marginally better. Nayak et al. (1976) have reported that chronic cocaine administration to rats (20 mg/kg, s.c., b.i.d.) reduced the uptake into the brain of a challenge dose of cocaine and increased the $t_{1/2}$; these authors concluded that appreciable sequestration into fat depots was a significant factor in this phenomenon. Reith et al. (1987) have examined the effects of intermittent and continuous cocaine administration on both the behavioral responses and plasma/brain levels of a subsequent cocaine challenge. Interestingly, these authors found that intermittent administration for 18 days *sensitized* the animals (mice) to the challenge dose, whereas continuous administration of the same total dose caused tolerance. They also found no significant differences in brain and plasma levels of cocaine between the two groups, nor was there any significant difference in the plasma levels of benzoylecgonine. However, in animals administered cocaine intermittently for 2 or 3 days, the challenge dose of cocaine produced a greater behavioral response (sensitization), which was associated with a higher brain level of cocaine. The mechanism of this latter phenomenon was not determined.

COCAINE METABOLISM AND CLEARANCE

Cocaine metabolism in man and animals is generally well understood. The major metabolites in man include benzoylecgonine, ecgonine methylester, and ecgonine. Since <5% of the parent drug is excreted in the urine, metabolism is clearly an important factor in terminating cocaine's actions. Cocaine has two ester linkages that are suitable substrates for the highly active intracellular and extracellular esterases (e.g., pseudocholinesterase). It also should be noted that the cleavage of the methylester linkage to yield benzoylecgonine may occur nonenzymatically in both plasma and urine (Fletcher & Hancock, 1981). This nonenzymatic cleavage increases with increasing pH, a factor of some concern since the organic extraction of cocaine from tissue samples or biological fluids is frequently performed at alkaline pH. The $t_{1/2}$ for cocaine in human plasma is approximately 1 hour, but the variation in $t_{1/2}$ is large. For example, Javaid et al. (1978) reported that $t_{1/2}$ varied from 40 to 91 minutes. The reasons for such variations in clearance are not known, but it is of interest to speculate that they may relate to individual variations in plasma cholinesterase activity. Such variations, which are important in determining sensitivity to succinyl-choline, are quantified in terms of plasma activity to hydrolyze dibucaine (yielding the dibucaine number). It has been suggested that individuals with low dibucaine numbers should metabolize cocaine more slowly than those with high numbers. Some in vitro data support this view (Stewart et al., 1979); the question that remains unanswered is whether individual variations in metabolism impact upon the pattern of drug administration.

It is noteworthy that, unlike cocaine, amphetamine is not extensively metabolized by humans and clearance occurs largely by excretion. Thus, the substitution of amphetamine for cocaine (which from the behavioral perspective may go unnoticed by the cocaine abuser) could result in a toxic crisis if the amphetamine were used in a manner similar to that of cocaine.

There is some suggestion in the clinical literature that both the route and dose of cocaine administration may affect plasma half-life. Wilkinson et al. (1980) reported $t_{1/2}$ values from oral and nasal administration of 48 and 75 minutes, respectively. Jeffcoat et al. (1989), studying cocaine disposition using $[4 - {}^3H]$ cocaine HCl, reported that the plasma elimination $t_{1/2}$ for intranasal, IV, and smoke inhalation was 78, 78, and 56 minutes, respectively. Using a somewhat different kinetic model, Barnett et al. (1981) recalculated the data of Wilkinson and determined $t_{1/2}$ values of 59 (p.o.) and 74 (n.t.) minutes. Regardless of the calculation, the sample size was too small to determine whether such differences are significant but the possibility that they are real should not be ignored. Barnett et al. (1981), in a study of four subjects receiving IV doses of cocaine, suggested that the biological or terminal phase $t_{1/2}$ could best be expressed in terms of a linear equation ($t_{1/2} = 13.5 \pm 24.5$ D) where $t_{1/2}$ is given in minutes and D is the dose in mg/kg over the range of 1 to 3 mg/kg. These authors argued that when relatively large doses of cocaine (e.g., 3 mg/kg) are administered, metabolism may reach saturation. The "apparent" dose dependency of cocaine's rate of disappearance was examined over the range of 1 to 4 mg/kg in sheep by Khan et al. (1987). These authors noted some tendency toward a decreased rate of clearance with an increasing dose, but the changes were not large or significant. Interpretation of these results in clinical terms is complicated by the fact that clearance in sheep (291 ml/min/kg) is 4 times greater than cardiac output (76 ml/min/kg). This wide discrepancy between clearance and cardiac output is not seen in other animal species such as rats, dogs, and monkeys (Misra, 1976) nor is it seen in man (Fischman & Schuster, 1982). Khan et al. (1987) argued that the discrepancy in sheep is probably associated with a significant pulmonary first-pass effect.

As might be expected, the rate of disappearance of cocaine from plasma in animals is faster than generally reported in humans. Benuck et al. (1987) found that in mice (female, BALB/cBy) the $t_{1/2}$ for both plasma and brain cocaine after i.p. injection was 16 minutes. In this study the $t_{1/2}$ did not show dose dependence over the range examined (10 and 25 mg/kg). The only metabolite examined was benzoylecgonine. Levels in the brain were too low for kinetic evaluation. In plasma the $t_{1/2}$ for benzoylecgonine, 62 minutes, was significantly greater than that for cocaine. Nayak et al. (1976) examined the rate of cocaine disappearance from rat brain and plasma after the IV administration of 8 mg/kg. The approximate half-lives were 0.4 (brain) and 0.3 (plasma) hours. These relatively rapid rates contrast with those for cocaine metabolites. Thus, benzoylecgonine and ecgonine show $t_{1/2}$ values in the brain of 1.3 and 7.8 hours, respectively, and in plasma of 0.8 and 3.8 hours, respectively (Misra et al., 1974, 1975). The study of Nayak et al. (1976) is informative in that data on the distribution of cocaine in 11 different tissues is provided for both acute and chronic s.c. administration. With chronic cocaine administration, there is some redistribution in the time of peak levels, so that proportionally more cocaine is found in lung and fat. The urinary and fecal excretion of cocaine were examined in the same acute/chronic paradigm. As noted elsewhere in this chapter, only a small amount (in this case <2%) of cocaine was excreted. There was no increase in the amount of parent compound excreted with chronic administration, nor was there a significant difference in urinary excretion of cocaine metabolites (cumulative total, 49.3% [acute] versus 51.6% [chronic]). However, fecal excretion of metabolites did increase 62% (cumulative total, 22.1%

[acute] versus 35.9% [chronic]). The main metabolites found in urine were benzoylecgonine, benzoylnorecgonine (derived from norcocaine), ecgonine methylester, and ecgonine; this pattern of metabolism is similar to that found clinically.

The examination of urinary cocaine metabolites is forensically as well as scientifically interesting. Since the amounts of un-metabolized cocaine excreted are small, the presence of persistent cocaine metabolites such as benzoylecgonine is used as proof of a "positive" urine test. Baselt and Chang (1987) examined the appear-ance of urinary metabolites from a single oral dose of 25 mg. The cocaine was administered in a caffeine-free soda; the subject re-ported only mild effects. Peak cocaine levels in urine (as determined by GC/MS) were found 1 hour after administration (269 ng/ml); urinary cocaine levels dropped to 23 ng/ml by 6 hours; and no urinary cocaine was detected at 12 hours after administration. In contrast, benzoylecgonine levels peaked at 12 hours after adminis-tration (7,940 ng/ml), and detectable levels were still present 72 hours after administration (58 ng/ml). Ambre (1985) has reviewed the literature on the urinary excretion of cocaine and metabolites; some details of this review will be recounted here. Fish and Wilson (1969) recovered (in urine) 44% of the cocaine administered as ben-zoylecgonine, 1% to 8% as ecgonine and 2% to 3% as cocaine. Ambre (1985) examined the urinary metabolites in four healthy co-caine users after the IV and n.t. administration of cocaine at 16, 32, 64, and 96 mg doses. The data showed that the urinary concentra-tions of ecgonine methyl ester are generally comparable to those of benzoylecgonine, with 26% to 60% of the total dose administered excreted as ecgonine methyl ester (its half-life was 4.2 hours com-pared to 5.1 hours for benzoylecgonine). Inaba et al. (1978) exam-ined the urinary excretion of ^{14}C-cocaine. Benzoylecgonine accounted for 50% to 60% of urinary radioactivity, whereas ecgonine methyl ester and cocaine accounted for 41% and 3%, re-spectively. A recent study by Jeffcoat et al. (1989) measured the urinary excretion products of ^{3}H-cocaine after IV, intranasal, and smoke inhalation in recreational users. Benzoylecgonine accounted for approximately 40% of the urinary radioactivity measured after IV and intranasal routes ($N = 4$), but only 26% after smoke inhala-tion ($N = 6$). In contrast, the urinary excretions of cocaine (>1%), ecgonine (>3%), and ecgonine methyl ester (18%–22%) were approximately equivalent regardless of the route of administration. Fecal excretion was minor but higher after smoke inhalation compared to intranasal or IV administration. From his survey of the literature and reexamination of his own data, Ambre (1985) constructed a nomogram relating urinary benzoylecgonine concentrations to the size and time interval since the last cocaine dose. Finally, it should be noted that in addition to the major urinary metabolites, a number of minor metabolites have been identified. These include the arylhydroxy metabolites (e.g., 2'-hydroxycocaine) and the hydroxymethoxybenzoylmethylecgonines (e.g., 4'-hydroxy-3-methoxybenzoylecgonine methyl ester) (Smith, 1984; Smith et al., 1984).

COCAINE TOXICITY

The increasing abuse of cocaine has led to an increasing number of cocaine-related deaths (e.g., Finkle & McCloskey, 1978; Mittleman & Wetli, 1984; Poklis et al., 1985; Spiehler & Reed, 1985; Wetli & Fishbain, 1985; Winek et al., 1987). The data obtained from postmortem analysis allow us to bracket the toxic plasma and brain concentrations of cocaine and its metabolites. Wetli and Fishbain (1985) found that the blood concentration of cocaine ranged from 140 to 960 ng/ml in 7 social-recreational users who died unexpectedly. This dose range is not significantly greater than the levels reported for the pharmacokinetic studies discussed in previous sections. Spiehler and Reed (1985) reported on 37 cases of cocaine overdose. The average blood concentration was 4,600 ng/ml with a range of 40 to 31,000 ng/ml. The average blood benzoylecgonine concentration was 7,900 ng/ml, with a range of 700 to 20,000 ng/ml. The average brain cocaine and benzoylecgonine concentrations were 13,300 and 2,900 ng/ml, respectively. The brain cocaine concentrations ranged from 170 to 31,400 ng/ml. These 37 cases were compared to 46 cases in which cocaine was present but incidental to the cause of death. The ratio of cocaine/benzoylecgonine in the brain and blood of the toxic cases (14.7 and 0.64, respectively) was clearly different from the ratios found in the incidental cases (0.87 [brain] and 0.27 [blood]). In the toxic cases, the brain/blood ratios were 9.6 and 0.36 for cocaine and benzoylecgonine, respectively, compared with 2.5 and 1.4 in the incidental cases. The ratios in the toxic studies are consistent with those reported for animal studies, soon after cocaine administration. The higher ratio for benzoylecgonine in the incidental cases is consistent with the tissue accumulation and persistence of cocaine metabolites. The doses associated with the plasma levels discussed above are difficult to determine because of the wide variability among individuals for metabolism of cocaine (Jones, 1984). Acute administration of doses of 100–300 mg of cocaine in human subjects appear to have little or no untoward effect (Jones, 1984). However, there have been reports of deaths after doses as small as 20 mg of cocaine in patients with histories of congenital blood and liver esterase deficiency (Cohen, 1985). The average lethal dose of cocaine has been estimated to be about 1.2 gm (Arena, 1974).

Cocaine-related deaths are frequently preceded by hyperexia, convulsions, excited delirium, and shock (Jaffe, 1985; Wetli & Wright, 1979). Cocaine can cause death by a variety of mechanisms such as ventricular fibrillation, myocardial infarction, apnea, pulmonary edema, convulsion, and cerebral hemorrhages (Cregler & Mark, 1986). Reports of specific cardiac toxicity are increasingly common (e.g., Allred & Evver, 1981; Coleman et al., 1982; Cregler & Mark, 1985; Mathias, 1986; Nanji & Filipenko, 1984; Wiener et al., 1986). Physical complications from cocaine are associated with all routes of administration and are not only limited to "massive doses." For example, in one patient a cardiac arrhythmia occurred after intravenous administration of 140 mg and in another an acute myocardial infarction occurred after 0.25 g of cocaine IV (Isner et al., 1986).

There have also been reports on the effects of chronic cocaine administration in humans and animals. The drug is particularly toxic in situations of free availability as demonstrated by Johanson et al. (1984), who exposed two rhesus monkeys to continuous access to cocaine. These monkeys took the drug in doses of 20–100 mg kg/day. Both animals died 3–5 days after initiating the experiment. In humans, chronic cocaine administration has been reported to induce psychoses, depression, convulsions, and death (Fischman, 1984). Complications from chronic cocaine abuse in humans have been reported to occur at doses as low as 25 mg (Lowenstein, 1987).

SUMMARY

Despite the variation in some reports, the following are general conclusions regarding the pharmacokinetics of cocaine in humans:

1. Cocaine has a rapid initial distribution phase
2. The bioavailability of cocaine ranges from 30% to 100% and is dependent upon route of administration
3. Cocaine's principal route of elimination is metabolism by hydrolytic pathways in plasma and the liver; its clearance is primarily nonrenal
4. The primary urinary metabolites are benzoylecgonine, ecgonine methyl ester, and ecgonine, and less than 5% of cocaine is excreted unchanged.

Finally, the administration of cocaine by intravenous injection, nasal insufflation (snorting), or smoke inhalation produces levels of cocaine in excess of the benchmark concentration (150 mg/ml) needed to facilitate reinforcement.

REFERENCES

Allred, R. J. & Evver, S. (1981) Fatal pulmonary edema following intravenous "freebase" cocaine use. *Ann. Emerg. Med.* 10:441–442.

Ambre, J. (1985) The urinary excretion of cocaine and metabolites in humans: A kinetic analysis of published data. *J. Anal. Toxicol.* 9:241–245.

Ambre, J. J., Ruo, J. H., Smith, G. L., Backer, D. & Smith, C. M. (1982) Ecgonine methyl ester, a major metabolite of cocaine. *J. Anal. Toxicol.* 626–629.

Arena, J. M. (1974) *Poisoning: Toxicology symptoms treatment.* Springfield, Ill.: Charles C. Thomas, 375.

Barnett, G., Hawks, R. & Resnick, R. (1981) Cocaine pharmacokinetics in humans. *J. Ethnopharmacol.* 3:353–366.

Baselt, R. C. & Chang, R. (1987) Urinary excretion of cocaine and benzoylecgonine following oral ingestion in a single subject. *J. Anal. Toxicol.* 11: 81–82.

Benuck, M., Lajtha, A. & Reith, M.E.A. (1987) Pharmacokinetics of systemically administered cocaine and locomotor stimulation in mice. *J. Pharmacol. Exp. Ther.* 243:144–149.

Broekkamp, C. L., LePichon, M. & Lloyd, K. G. (1984) Akinesia after locally applied morphine near the nucleus raphé pontis of the rat. *Neurosci. Lett.* 50:313–318.

Chow, M. J., Ambre, J. J., Ruo, J. H., Tsuen, I. H., Atkinson, A. J., Bowsher, D. J. & Fischman, M. W. (1985) Kinetics of cocaine distribution, elimination and chronotropic effects. *Clin. Pharmacol. Ther.* 38:318–324.

Cohen, S. (1985) Reinforcement and rapid delivery systems: Understanding adverse consequences of cocaine. In: Kozel, N. J. & Adams, E. H. (Eds.), *Cocaine use in America: Epidemiologic and clinical perspectives*. NIDA Research Monograph 61, DHHS pub. no. (ADM) 85-1414. Washington, D.C.: Government Printing Office, 151–157.

Coleman, D. L., Ross, T. F. & Naughton, J. L. (1982) Myocardial ischemia and infarction related to recreational cocaine use. *West. J. Med.* 136 (5):444–446.

Cregler, L. L. & Mark, H. (1985) Relation of acute myocardial infarction to cocaine abuse. *Am. J. Cardiol.* 56: 794.

Cregler, L. L. & Mark, H. (1986) Medical complications of cocaine abuse. *N. Engl. J. Med.* 315:1495–1500.

Finkle, B. S. & McCloskey, K. L. (1978) The forensic toxicology of cocaine. *J. Forensic Sci.* 23:173–189.

Fischman, M. W. (1984) The behavioral pharmacology of cocaine in humans. In: Grabowski, J. (Ed.), *Cocaine: Pharmacology, effects, and treatment of abuse*, NIDA Research Monograph 50, DHHS publication no 84-1326. Washington, D.C.: U.S. Government Printing Office, 72–91.

Fischman, M. W. & Schuster, C. R. (1982) Cocaine self-administration in humans. *Fed. Proc.* 41:241–246.

Fish, F. & Wilson, W. D. C. (1969) Excretion of cocaine and its metabolites in man. *J. Pharm. Pharmacol.* 21:1355–1385.

Fletcher, S. M. & Hancock, V. S. (1981) Potential errors in benzoylecgonine and cocaine analysis. *J. Chromatogr.* 206(1):193–195.

Ford, R. D. & Balster, R. L. (1977) Reinforcing properties of intravenous procaine in rhesus monkeys. *Pharmacol. Biochem. Behav.* 6:289–296.

Grabowski, J. (1984) *Cocaine: Pharmacology, effects, and treatment of abuse*. NIDA Research Monograph 50, DHHS pub. no. (ADM) 24-1326. Washington, D.C.: Government Printing Office.

Hammerbeck, D. M. & Mitchell, C. L. (1978) The reinforcing properties of procaine and d-amphetamine compared in rhesus monkeys. *J. Pharmacol. Exp. Ther.* 204:558–569.

Horne, A. S., Coyle, J. T. & Snyder, S. H. (1971) Catecholamine uptake by synaptosomes from rat brain. Structure-activity relationships of drugs with different effects on dopamine and norepinephrine neurons. *Mol. Pharmacol.* 7:66–80.

Inaba, T., Stewart, D. J. & Kalow W. (1978) Metabolism of cocaine in man. *Clin. Pharmacol. Ther.* 23:547–552.

Isner, J. M., Estes, M. & Thompson, P. (1986) Acute cardiac events temporarily related to cocaine abuse. *N. Engl. J. Med.* 315:1438–1443.

Jaffe, J. H. (1985) Drug addiction and drug abuse. In: Gilman, A. G., Goodman, L. S., Rall, T. W. & Murad, F. (Eds.), *The pharmacological basis of therapeutics* (7th ed.). New York: Macmillan, 500–554.

Jatlow, P. & Bailey, D. (1975) Gas chromatographic analysis for cocaine in human plasma with use of a nitrogen detector. *Clin. Chem.* 21:1918–1921.

Javaid, J. I., Fischman, M. W., Schuster, C. R., Dekirmenjiian, H. & Davis, J. M. (1978) Cocaine plasma concentration: Relation to physiological and subjective effects in human. *Science* 202:227–228.

Javaid, J. I., Musa, M. N., Fischman, M., Schuster, C. R. & Davis, J. M. (1983) Kinetics of cocaine in humans after intravenous and intranasal administration. *Biopharm. Drug Disp.* 4:9–18.

Jeffcoat, A. R., Perez-Reyes, M., Hill, J. M., Sadler, B. M. & Cook, C. E. (1989) Cocaine disposition in humans after intravenous injection, nasal insufflation (snorting), or smoking. *Drug Metab. Disp.* 17:153–159.

Jeri, F. R., Sanchez, C., Del Pozo, T. & Fernandez, M. (1978) The syndrome of coca paste. *J. Psychedel. Drugs* 10(4):361–370.

Johanson, C. E. (1984) Assessment of the dependence potential of cocaine in animals. In: Grabowski, S. (Ed.), *Cocaine: Pharmacology, effects, and treatment of abuse,* NIDA Research Monograph 50, DHHS pub. no. (ADM) 84-1326. Washington, D.C.: Government Printing Office, 54–71.

Khan, M., Gupta, P. K., Cristie, R., Nangia, A., Winter, H., Lam, F. C. & Perrier, D. G. (1987) Determination of pharmacokinetics of cocaine in sheep by liquid chromatography. *J. Pharm. Sci.* 76:39–43.

Koob, G. F., Vaccasina, F. J., Amalric, M. & Swederlow, N. K. (1987) Neural substrates for cocaine and opiate reinforcement. In: Fischer, S., Raskin, A. & Uklenhuth, E. H. (Eds.), *Cocaine: Clinical and biobehavioral aspects.* New York: Oxford University Press, 80–108.

Kozel, N. J. & Adams, E. H. (1985) *Cocaine use in America: Epidemiologic and clinical perspectives.* NIDA Research Monograph 61, DHHS pub. no. (ADM) 85-1414. Washington, D.C.: Government Printing Office.

Lowenstein, D., Massa, S. & Rowbotham, M. C. (1987) Acute neurologic and psychiatric complications associated with cocaine abuse. *Am. J. Med.* 83:-841–846.

Mathias, D. W. (1986) Cocaine-associated myocardial ischemia. *Am. J. Med.* 81:675–678.

Misra, A. L. (1976) Disposition and biotransformation of cocaine. In: Mulé, S. J. (Ed.), *Cocaine: Chemical, biological, clinical, social and treatment aspects.* Cleveland: CRC Press, 73–90.

Misra, A. L., Nayak, P. K., Bloch, R. & Mulé, S. J. (1975) Estimation and disposition of [^{3}H]benzoylecgonine and pharmacological activity of some cocaine metabolites. *J. Pharm. Pharmacol.* 27:784–786.

Misra, A. L., Nayak, P. K., Patel, M. N., Vadlamani, N. L. & Mulé, S. J. (1974) Identification of norcocaine as a metabolite of [^{3}H]-cocaine in rat brain. *Experientia* (Basel) 30:1312–1314.

Mittleman, E. & Wetli, C. V. (1984) Death caused by recreational cocaine use. *JAMA* 252(14):1988–1993.

Nanji, M. B. & Filipenko, J. D. (1984) Asystole and ventricular fibrillation associated with cocaine intoxication. *Chest* 85:132–133.

Nayak, P. K., Misra, A. L. & Mulé, S. J. (1976) Physiological disposition and biotransformation of [3H]cocaine in acutely and chronically treated rats. *J. Pharmacol. Exp. Ther.* 196:556–559.

Paly, D., Jatlow, P., Van Dyke, C., Jeri, R. & Byck, R. (1982) Plasma cocaine concentrations during cocaine paste smoking. *Life Sci.* 30(9):731–738.

Poklis, A., Mackell, M. A. & Graham, M. (1985) Disposition of cocaine in fatal poisoning in man. *J. Anal. Toxicol.* 9:227–229.

Reith, M. E. A., Benuck, M. & Lajtha, A. (1987) Cocaine disposition in the brain after continuous or intermittent treatment and locomotor stimulation in mice. *J. Pharmacol. Exp. Ther.* 243:281–288.

Reith, M. E. A., Meisler, B. E. & Lajtha, A. (1985) Locomotor effects of cocaine, cocaine cogeners, and local anesthetics in mice. *Pharmacol. Biochem. Behav.* 23:831–836.

Ritchie, J. M. & Greene, M. N. (1980) Local anesthetics. In: Gilman, A. G. & Goodman, L. S. (Eds.), *The pharmacological basis of therapeutics.* New York: Macmillan, 300–320.

Ritz, M. C., Lamb, R. J., Goldberg, S. R. & Kuhar, M. J. (1987) Cocaine receptors on dopamine transporters are related to self-administration of cocaine. *Science* 237:1219–1222.

Siegel, R. K. (1984) The changing patterns of cocaine use: Longitudinal observations, consequences, and treatment. In: Grabowski, J. (Ed.), *Cocaine: Pharmacology, effects, and treatment of abuse.* NIDA Research Monograph 50, DHHS pub. no. (ADM) 84-1326. Washington, D.C.: Government Printing Office, 92-110.

Smith, R. M. (1984) Arylhydroxy metabolites of cocaine in the urine of cocaine users. *J. Anal. Toxicol.* 8:35–37.

Smith, R. M., Poquette, M. A. & Smith, P. J. (1984) Hydroxymethoxybenzoylmethylecgonines: New metabolites of cocaine from human urine. *J. Anal. Toxicol.* 8:29–34.

Spiehler, V. R. & Reed, D. (1985) Brain concentrations of cocaine and benzoylecgonine in fatal cases. *J. Forensic Sci.* 30:1003–1011.

Stewart, D. J., Inbaba, T., Lucassen, M. & Kalow, W. (1979) Cocaine metabolism: Cocaine and norcocaine hydrolysis by liver and serum esterases. *Clin. Pharmacol. Ther.* 25:464–468.

Van Dyke, C. & Byck, R. (1982) Cocaine. *Sci. Am.* 246:128–134.

Van Dyke, C., Jatlow, P., Barash, P. G. & Byck, R. (1978) Oral cocaine: Plasma concentrations and central effects. *Science* 100:211–213.

Wetli, C. V. & Fishbain, D. A. (1985) Cocaine-induced psychosis and sudden death in recreational cocaine users. *J. Forensic Sci.* 30(3):873–880.

Wetli, C. V. & Wright, R. K. (1979) Deaths caused by recreational cocaine use. *JAMA* 241:2519–2522.

Wiener, R. S., Lockhart, J. T. & Schwartz, R. G. (1986) Dilated cardiomyopathy and cocaine abuse. *Am. J. Med.* 81:699–701.

Wilkinson, P., Van Dyke, C., Jatlow, P., Brash, P. & Byck, R. (1980) Intranasal and oral cocaine kinetics. *Clin. Pharmacol. Ther.* 27(3):386–394.

Winek, C. L., Wahba, W. W., Rozin, L. & Janssen, J. K. (1987) An unusually high blood cocaine concentration in a fatal case. *J. Anal. Toxicol.* 11:43–46.

7

Medical, Endocrinological, and Pharmacological Aspects of Cocaine Addiction

Charles A. Dackis and Mark S. Gold

The reinforcing and toxic actions of cocaine have been linked to its sympathomimetic effects (Jatlow, 1987). The toxic properties and their medical consequences have mainly been linked to cocaine's ability to block norepinephrine reuptake (Wilkerson, 1988). Its reinforcing and addicting properties, on the other hand, have been linked to its ability to block the dopamine reuptake. The effects of cocaine on the dopamine system have led to the "dopamine depletion hypothesis" as the mechanism accounting for cocaine craving. In this chapter we will review the most frequent medical complications associated with cocaine use, the nature of dopamine changes occurring in the brain of the cocaine addict, and their implications with respect to pharmacological interventions.

MEDICAL CONSEQUENCES OF COCAINE USE

Although its mythology once portrayed a safe and harmless drug, we now know that cocaine produces numerous medical complications (Cregler & Mark, 1986) and is probably a more toxic substance than heroin (Bozarth & Wise, 1985). Many complications from cocaine can be traced to its direct actions in the tissue and to its route of administration. Intranasal use is associated with sinusitis, rhinitis, ethmoiditis, perforated nasal septum, optic neuropathies, and nosebleeds (MacFarland et al., 1989). Intrapulmonary

135

(smoking "freebase" or "crack" preparations) administration can lead to pneumothorax and pneumomediastinum from the forced inhalation of the drug (Hunter et al., 1986), as well as to damage of pulmonary function (Itkonen et al., 1984; Weiss et al., 1981). Intravenous use can lead to AIDS, hepatitis, endocarditis, pneumonia, vasculopathies, sepsis, and meningitis from the use of contaminated needles (Chaisson et al., 1989). The intravenous routes can also lead to embolic complication from injection of crystals of other nonsoluble material. The intravenous and pulmonary routes of administration lead to the most severe forms of addiction resulting from the prompt delivery of cocaine to the brain.

Other effects of cocaine occur independently of the route of administration and result from direct toxic or pharmacological actions on organ systems. Systemic effects of acute intoxication include hypertension, tachycardia, hyperglycemia, and hyperthermia. Death by hyperthermia has been described (Wetli, 1981), as has hypertension to the point of aortic rupture (Barth et al., 1986) and cerebral hemorrhage (Schwartz & Cohen, 1984). Many systemic effects result from acute autonomic arousal, probably mediated largely through central and peripheral norepinephrine stimulation.

Numerous other medical complications have been described in chronic cocaine abusers. Patients frequently complain of malaise, decreased energy, sexual dysfunction, depression, headaches, irritability, and sleep problems (Washton & Gold, 1984). Spontaneous abortions are common when cocaine is used during pregnancy, and the neurologic behavior of the newborn can be adversely affected (Chasnoff et al., 1985). In addition, because of the marked adulteration that cocaine undergoes (average purity of 40%), one needs to consider the toxic properties of the adulterant used in cocaine trafficking (Shannon, 1988). Of particular concern are adulteration with anesthetics, stimulants, and toxins, since some of the compounds can act synergistically with cocaine to increase its toxicity and lethality. Other substances used as adulterants, such as phenylpropanolamine and amphetamine, exert direct toxic effects on various organ systems (Salanova & Taubner, 1984). Emergency room visits by patients using cocaine are currently surging (Schuster, 1987; Washton & Gold, 1984). Therefore, the myth of medical safety that once encouraged first time users is gradually fading, as it has during past cocaine epidemics.

Cardiovascular Consequences

Pharmacological actions of cocaine account for some of the cardio-vascular events reported in cocaine abusers. The sympathomimetic action, for example, can lead to vasoconstriction and increases in heart rate and blood pressure (Isner et al., 1986; Resnick et al., 1977). The increase in blood pressure can, in turn, generate a higher incidence of hemorrhages, a higher load of activity on the heart, and ischemia secondary to vasoconstriction (Hueter, 1989). Rupture of the aorta in a healthy patient smoking freebase cocaine secondary to an increase in blood pressure has also been reported (Barth et al., 1986).

There have been several reports of acute myocardial infarction related to cocaine abuse in patients who had persistent heart disease, as well as in those with no previous history of heart disease (Duke, 1986; Howard et al., 1985; Isner et al., 1986). Myocardial infarction in the presence of normal coronary arteries was explained by vaso-constriction of the coronary arteries secondary to cocaine, whereas vasospasm from cocaine, in addition to increased systolic blood pressure and myocardial oxygen demand, could explain the exacer-bation of preexisting coronary disease (Simpson & Edwards, 1986). Myocardial infarctions have been reported to occur with all routes of cocaine administration.

Several arrhythmias have been associated with cocaine abuse, in-cluding ventricular premature contractions, ventricular tachycardia, and ventricular fibrillations (Bates, 1988; Cregler & Mark, 1986). These arrhythmogenic effects probably result from the potentiation by cocaine of catecholamines, mainly norepinephrine, in the heart.

Another mechanism that may contribute to the cardiotoxicity of cocaine is its potentiation of platelet aggregation, which would fa-vor the occurrence of platelet thrombi (Heuter, 1989; Togna et al., 1985). In fact, autopsies performed in cases of cocaine-related myo-cardial infarction reported vessel obstruction due to platelet throm-bosis (Simpson & Edwards, 1986). In addition, it has also been postulated that cocaine favors the development of arteriosclerosis (Ring & Butman, 1986). The atherogenic effect of cocaine appears to be due to damage of the arterial wall secondary to increases in blood pressure and heart rate (Langner et al., 1988). Because of all of these effects, cocaine abuse "might have to be viewed as a possible risk factor for coronary disease" (Hueter, 1989). Treatment of the cardiac complications from cocaine should be managed as other cardiac events. Cardiac toxicity from acute cocaine has been treated successfully with propranolol and has recently been reported to respond to the calcium channel blocker, nitrendipine (Nahas et al., 1985).

Obstetrical, Neonatal, and Developmental Complications

Because of the widespread abuse of cocaine among women of reproductive age, the effects of cocaine abuse on pregnancy are important. Indeed, cocaine use in pregnancy is associated with a higher rate of spontaneous abortions, as well as of abruptio placentae (Bates, 1988). These effects have been explained in part by the hypertension and vasoconstriction of placental vessels induced by cocaine as a consequence of its ability to increase norepinephrine at the synaptic cleft (Chasnoff et al., 1985). Vasoconstriction in the uterine vascular bed with reduction in uterine blood flow from cocaine (Woods et al., 1987) could impair fetal homeostasis, which may explain some of the higher rates of congenital malformation, perinatal mortality, and neuroimpairment of infants born to mothers who abuse cocaine. However, some of these abnormalities could also be due to the direct effects of cocaine on the fetus (Geggel et al., 1989). Indeed, studies with animals have demonstrated that cocaine not only decreases uterine blood flow, but also passes into the fetal circulation (Moore et al., 1986). Furthermore, neither the fetus nor the newborn can metabolize cocaine as efficiently as the adult does, extending the duration of exposure to cocaine and to its active metabolites. Though several studies have reported on the debilitative effects of cocaine exposure during pregnancy on the newborn (Chasnoff et al., 1985), there is very little information about its teratogenecity or about its repercussions later during development. A recent study done in a group of 70 infants born to mothers who had abused cocaine during pregnancy reported decreased head circumference in these babies compared to match controls (MacGregor et al., 1987).

Use of cocaine during pregnancy has been associated with skull

defects (Bingol et al., 1987; Chasnoff et al., 1989) and growth retar-
dation. Animal studies of cocaine teratology have documented both
an increase in fetal fatality when cocaine is administered during
pregnancy (Dow Edwards, 1988) and impaired learning processes
and behavior in some of the surviving animals (Smith et al., 1989;
Spear et al., 1987). Similarly, human studies have documented neurobehavioral deficiencies in newborn babies when the mothers were
exposed to cocaine during the first trimester (Chasnoff et al., 1989).

Respiratory Complications

Intranasal use of cocaine produces vasoconstriction associated with
sinusitis, rhinitis, ethmoiditis, perforated nostril septum, and nose
bleeds. Respiratory problems associated with cocaine abuse have
also been described. The most common presentation is sore throat,
chest pain, and black or bloody sputum (Nakamura & Nogvch,
1981; Vilensky, 1982). Complications are more frequent in individuals who freebase cocaine (Bates, 1988). Both pneumomediastinum
and pneumopericardium have been associated with cocaine inhalation, secondary to exaggerated inspiratory efforts when performing
a Valsalva's maneuver to inhale the cocaine (Aroesty et al., 1986;
Schweitzer, 1986). Inhalation of freebase cocaine has also been associated with derangements in gas exchange by the lungs (Itkonen et
al., 1984). Smoking cocaine can induce changes in pulmonary function that suggest irritant effects on both large and small airways
(Tashkin et al., 1987). In one case, cocaine inhalation produced a
hypersensitivity lung reaction with pulmonary infiltrates, fever, and
bronchospasms (Weiss et al., 1981). Lung damage and pulmonary
edema have also been reported in freebasers. Finally, cocaine can
induce respiratory failure leading to death. The latter appears to be
an effect of cocaine on the central nervous system.
     The mechanisms underlying the pathological effects of cocaine
on the lung are unclear. Some of them could relate to the sympathomimetic and anesthetic properties of cocaine. Sympathomimetic effects due to the blockade of uptake of neurotransmitters could lead
to an excess of neurotransmitters at the receptor site. Anesthetic
properties, on the other hand, could prevent some of the physiological homeostatic responses of the lung.

Brain Consequences

Cocaine abuse has been associated with neurological and psychiatric symptoms. The effects of cocaine on the brain range from mild agitation to seizures, convulsions, and death (Cregler & Mark, 1986; Gawin, 1988; Satel & Gawin, 1989). The toxic actions of cocaine in the brain can be multiple: Some of these are related to the vasoactive properties of cocaine; more specifically, cocaine has been associated with cerebral infarctions, cerebral hemorrhage, and stroke (Cregler & Mark, 1987; Nolte & Gelman, 1989; Wojak & Flamm, 1987). Ischemic events have been reported in patients who complain of paresis and paralysis. Abnormalities in vascular and cerebral vessels after cocaine abuse have been demonstrated with measurements of cerebral blood flow in cocaine abusers (Volkow et al., 1988). Cerebral infarction was also reported in a newborn from a cocaine-abusing mother (Chasnoff et al., 1986). One possible explanation for the cerebral vasoconstriction secondary to cocaine abuse could be related to potentiation of serotonin by cocaine, since serotonin is the most potent vasoconstrictor amine in cerebral circulation (Edvenson & MacKinzie, 1976).

Cocaine abuse has also been associated with cerebral vasculitis in a patient who presented with neurological symptoms characterized by cranial nerve paralysis as well as a flaccid left-sided hemiparesis (Khaye & Fainstadt, 1987). It is possible that vasculitis may be an unrecognized complication of cocaine, since vasculitis has been demonstrated in association with intravenous amphetamine use, which shares many of the properties of cocaine. The pathogenesis of vasculitis from cocaine and amphetamine abuse remains unknown and could result from a reaction to impurities of administered drugs or from subarachnoid hemorrhage (Weingarten, 1988).

Respiratory failure is a cause of sudden death, and may result from the inhibition of medullary centers in the brain (Jonsson et al., 1983). Seizures are a frequent complication of cocaine use, and can occur after a single dose of the drug (Van Dyke & Byck, 1982). Lethal status epilepticus secondary to cocaine overdose has been reported (Myers & Earnest, 1984). Seizures induced by cocaine are increasingly likely with repeated exposure to the drug (Post et al., 1976). This phenomenon of sensitization, termed "kindling," may result from supersensitization of receptors in the brain, as discussed more extensively in the chapter by Swann. Since seizure disorders can be unmasked or induced by cocaine's "kindling" effect on the brain, the proper medical evaluation of these patients must rule out epilepsy.

The convulsions secondary to cocaine could relate directly to the action of cocaine on neuronal tissue. Indeed, in animals cocaine has been found to increase multiple unit activity of the reticular formation and to produce synchronization and an arousal effect on the EEG (Walla & Gershon, 1971). The EEG pattern and the cocaine-induced seizures resemble temporal lobe epilepsy (Van Dyke & Byck, 1977), in agreement with the high sensitivity of the temporal lobes to cocaine (Stevens et al., 1969). A report summarizing the most frequent neurological complications from cocaine seen in 196 emergency room visits in the years 1979 and 1986 included, in order of frequency, seizures, focal neurological symptoms and signs, headaches, and transient loss of consciousness (Rowbotham et al., 1987). Psychiatric symptoms secondary to cocaine abuse range from depression to psychoses (Post, 1975; Sherer, et al., 1988; Siegel, 1978) and are reviewed in the chapter by Gawin and Ellinwood.

ENDOCRINE EFFECTS

Thyroid Axis

The thyroid axis presents an interesting illustration of how clinical manifestations of cocaine use might parallel neurochemical alterations. Many clinical manifestations of cocaine intoxication are also found as signs and symptoms of hyperthyroidism. These include hypertension, hyperkinesis, diaphoresis, tachycardia, tremor, anxiety, and hyperthermia. Conversely, the cocaine "crash" (Dackis et al., 1985a; Gawin & Kleber, 1986) shares many signs and symptoms with the hypothyroid state, such as anergia, depression, bradykinesis, weight gain, and hypersomnia.

It is likely that cocaine intoxication is associated with thyroid axis activation. Monkeys treated with dextroamphetamine, which has neurochemical actions similar to those of cocaine, have elevated levels of thyroxine (T4) and thyroid-stimulating hormone (TSH)

(Morley et al., 1980), and rats treated with amphetamine are relatively hyperthyroid (Mantegazza et al., 1968). In addition, cocaine addicts have been found to have elevated T4 levels (Morley et al., 1980). We found that patients withdrawing from cocaine had normal T3, T4, and TSH levels, but showed markedly blunted TSH responses to thyrotropin-releasing hormone (TRH) infusions (Dackis et al., 1985a; Dackis et al., 1985b). This finding is consistent with receptor downregulation in response to chronic activation of the thyroid axis, and is a sign of compensated hyperthyroidism (Saberi & Utinger, 1983).

TRH is under stimulatory regulation by the catecholamines, and direct hypothalamic infusions of either dopamine or norepinephrine increase release of TRH (Reichlin, 1975). The acute stimulation of these neurotransmitter systems during cocaine intoxication would therefore explain hyperthyroid findings in animals, and compensated hyperthyroidism in our human study. Similarly, thyroid activation might contribute to certain signs and symptoms of cocaine intoxication. With the sudden withdrawal of cocaine, TRH stimulation would abruptly cease, and might even be diminished with the functional depletions of dopamine and norepinephrine. Reduced TRH stimulation would occur in the face of desensitized pituitary TRH receptors (Dackis et al., 1985a), leading to a relatively hypothyroid state. Since even mild forms of hypothyroidism have been shown to be associated with anergia and depressive symptoms (Gold et al., 1982), thyroid axis inhibition may contribute significantly to the cocaine crash.

Prolactin

Prolactin-secreting cells are tonically inhibited by dopamine (MacLeod, 1976) and stimulated by serotonin neurons (Meltzer et al., 1976). As we previously discussed in relation to dopamine depletion, cocaine addicts often have hyperprolactinemia during cocaine withdrawal (Dackis et al., 1984; Dackis et al., 1985b; Mendelson et al., 1988). Elevated prolactin can lead to gynecomastia and galactorrhea in cocaine abusers (Cocores et al., 1986) and might contribute to sexual dysfunction that frequently occurs in chronic cocaine abuse, including infertility, impotence, and amenorrhea (Meltzer et al., 1976). Sexual dysfunction in cocaine addicts might also be due to dopamine alterations, since this neurotransmitter system is involved in sexual reward (Cocores et al., 1986). Although cocaine initially stimulates sexual drive (Dimijian, 1974), chronic addicts often complain that satisfactory sexual performance and enjoyment decline over time and become difficult without concomitant cocaine use. Bromocriptine, which rapidly normalizes hyperprolactinemia and stimulates dopamine circuits (Siegel, 1982), also reverses sexual dysfunction in cocaine abusers (Cocores et al., 1986). Since hyperprolactinemia produced by cocaine might contribute to clinically significant sexual dysfunction in cocaine addicts, prolactin levels should be obtained in symptomatic patients and bromocriptine treatment can be considered.

Cortisol

The effects of cocaine on the hypothalamic-pituitary-adrenal (HPA) axis have been inadequately researched and are poorly understood. In animal studies, cocaine has been reported to cause adrenocortical hypertrophy (Kirkby & Petchkovsky, 1973) and to release cortisol in high doses (Post, 1981). Other central stimulants such as methylamphetamine (Checkley, 1978) and dextroamphetamine (Sachar et al., 1980) release cortisol in man through what appears to be an alpha-adrenergic mechanism (Rees et al., 1970). The possibility that cocaine also releases cortisol in humans has not been researched. Since the HPA axis appears to be under inhibitory norepinephrine (Jones et al., 1976) and excitatory serotonin (Meltzer et al., 1982) regulation, investigation into the effects of cocaine on this axis may provide further insight into current knowledge regarding its acute and chronic effects on these neurotransmitters (Gold et al., 1985).

There is compelling evidence, reviewed in previous chapters in this book, that cocaine's euphoria is due to the activation of brain pleasure centers and that the functioning of these centers depends on dopamine neurotransmission (Corbett & Wise, 1980; Goeders & Smith, 1983; Wise, 1978, 1984). Though acute cocaine administration will increase the concentration of dopamine in the synapse by blocking dopamine reuptake (Hurd & Ungerstedt, 1989; Ross & Renyi, 1966) chronic cocaine exposure will eventually lead to a functional depletion of dopamine systems (see Table 7.1). Indeed, increased dopamine receptor binding has been found in some brain regions of animals treated with acute and repeated doses of cocaine (Taylor et al., 1979; Trulson & Ulissey, 1986), as a compensatory response to functional dopamine depletion (Raff, 1976). Repeated cocaine administration also increases tyrosine hydroxylase activity (Patrick & Barchas, 1977; Trulson & Ulissey, 1986), indicating compensatory synthesis of the neurotransmitter.

PHARMACOLOGICAL TREATMENT OF COCAINE ADDICTION

Knowledge about cocaine-induced neurochemical disruptions can translate into formulation of effective pharmacological interventions. Cocaine abuse has clear biological components, and only recently have biological solutions been proposed in the form of medications to treat craving and withdrawal states (Dackis & Gold, 1985b; Gawin, 1988; O'Brien et al., 1988). A theory usually precedes and predicts an effective new treatment, as in the case of clonidine for opiate detoxification (Gold et al., 1978). In other cases, new treatments have been developed more serendipitously. In the following section we will describe the theoretical basis of our approach to the treatment of cocaine abuse.

We evaluated dopamine function in a group of chronic cocaine addicts by measuring serum prolactin levels, which were increased in both males (Dackis et al., 1984) and females (Dackis, Estroff & Gold, 1985) during the first week of cocaine abstinence. Since

TABLE 7.1
Cocaine Actions on Dopamine Neurons

Reuptake blockade (acute activation of DA neurotransmission)
   Increased DA binding sites (compensated depletion)
   Increased tyrosine hydroxylase activity (increased synthesis)
   Increased DA metabolism in the synapse (3-methoxytyramine)
   Intraneuronal DA metabolism (inhibition of DA vesicle binding)
   Decreased DA functional tone (elevated prolactin)
   Parkinsonian symptoms during cocaine withdrawal

---

prolactin is under inhibitory regulation by tuberoinfundibular dopamine neurons (MacLeod, 1976), elevated levels would be consistent with dopamine depletion. Cocores et al. (1986) also found prolactin elevations during cocaine withdrawal in several patients. Gawin and Kleber (1985) measured prolactin levels in male and female cocaine addicts and did not find hyperprolactinemia. Their sample was comprised of outpatients, however, making it difficult to control for factors that might affect prolactin secretion such as the use of other drugs, psychosocial stressors, sleep disruptions, and diet. In a recent inpatient study, Mendelson et al. (1988) replicated our finding of hyperprolactinemia.

The direct measurement of dopamine function in five hospitalized male cocaine addicts was recently reported by Extein et al. (1987). Compared with five age-matched controls, the cocaine patients had significant reductions in the dopamine metabolite homovanillic acid (HVA), when measured 30 days after their last dose of cocaine. Interestingly, HVA levels were not reduced during the first days of cocaine abstinence, suggesting that dopamine depletion evolved after cocaine abstinence began.

We hypothesized that the mechanism of dopamine depletion by cocaine involves chronic uptake blockade (Dackis & Gold, 1985a). After reuptake from the synapse, dopamine is normally stored in secretory vesicles and reutilized by the presynaptic neuron. Cocaine would prevent this "recycling" by blocking dopamine reuptake and thereby exposing released dopamine to synaptic metabolism by catechol-0-methyltransferase (COMT). Elevations of the synaptic dopamine metabolite 3-methoxytyramine have been measured after cocaine treatment (DiGiulio et al., 1971), and are consistent with this mechanism of dopamine depletion. Just as dopamine activation leads to euphoria, dopamine depletion could lead to craving.

DOPAMINE AND COCAINE CRAVING

Clinicians who treat cocaine abusers are well aware of the central role that craving plays in recidivism and the perpetuation of the addiction. Cocaine abuse begins with recreational use, and progresses gradually to a compulsive addiction that encompasses and dominates all aspects of the addict's life. Addicts become obsessed with the attainment of cocaine euphoria, and subject to irresistible craving. Euphoria and craving alternate repeatedly over time, forming a cycle of addiction that becomes increasingly entrenched and uncontrollable. Craving could represent a signal from the brain for more cocaine, which would temporarily correct the dopamine depletion by activating neurotransmission, only to set the stage for further depletion after the release dopamine is metabolized. This acute amelioration followed by subsequent exacerbation of dopamine depletion could contribute significantly to the neurochemistry of cocaine addiction. Furthermore, the dopamine depletion hypothesis led to our administration of bromocriptine, a dopamine agonist, to a number of cocaine addicts.

We have since reported rapid and dramatic anticraving efficacy in open trials (Dackis & Gold, 1985b; Dackis & Gold, 1985c; Dackis, Gold, et al., 1985), and in a double-blind, placebo-controlled study using a single dose of bromocriptine (Dackis et al., 1987). This finding has been replicated by three other groups in open (Extein et al., 1986) and double-blind studies (Jaffe, 1987; Tennant & Sagherian, 1987). To date, no negative studies using bromocriptine for cocaine craving or withdrawal have been reported. Increased postsynaptic dopamine receptor density, dopamine depletion, and hyperprolactinemia are effectively normalized by bromocriptine (Siegel, 1982), and its rapid and specific symptom reversal may directly result from the normalization of these neurochemical imbalances.

Tennant and Sagherian (1987) found bromocriptine to be effective, but encountered side effects using oral doses of 15 mg daily. We (Dackis & Gold, 1985b) and Extein (Extein et al., 1986) found that daily doses of 2–5 mg did not produce significant side effects and were effective in alleviating craving (see Table 7.2). Dopamine receptor supersensitivity (Taylor et al., 1979) could account for the incidence of side effects using normal doses of bromocriptine (Tennant & Sagherian, 1987), and for the extraordinarily low doses of bromocriptine that can be used effectively in cocaine patients. Tennant (1986) has also reported efficacy against cocaine craving and withdrawal with amantadine, which releases dopamine into the synapse, and with L-Dopa (Tennant, 1986), a precursor in the dopamine synthesis. The efficacy of these agents is consistent with the dopamine depletion hypothesis of cocaine craving and withdrawal.

We currently administer a 14-day course of bromocriptine in symptomatic cocaine-abusing patients (see Table 7.2). We have also reported rapid (2–5 days) antidepressant efficacy with bromocriptine in cocaine addicts, based on preliminary open studies (Dackis et al., 1986; Dackis & Gold, 1987). Maintenance bromocriptine treatment may be necessary if craving or depressive symptoms recur after the medication is discontinued. Further research should clarify the efficacy of bromocriptine and other dopamine agonist treatments, (Berger et al., 1989) and address specific treatment regimens.

Tricyclic antidepressants have also been reported to have efficacy in the treatment of cocaine withdrawal with beneficial effects occurring after several days or weeks (Gawin, 1988; Gawin & Kleber, 1984). It remains unclear whether the reported effectiveness repre-

TABLE 7.2

Bromocriptine Regimen for Cocaine Withdrawal

Day	Bromocriptine dose	Frequency
1	0.625 mg	t.i.d.
2	0.625 mg	t.i.d.
3	0.625 mg	q.i.d.
4	1.25 mg	b.i.d.
5	1.25 mg	t.i.d.
6	1.25 mg	t.i.d.
7	1.25 mg	t.i.d.
8	2.5 mg	t.i.d.
9	2.5 mg	t.i.d.
10	2.5 mg	t.i.d.
11	1.25 mg	t.i.d.
12	1.25 mg	b.i.d.
13	0.625 mg	b.i.d.
14	0.625 mg	b.i.d.
15	Discontinue bromocriptine	

NOTE: Titration of the dose is necessary, with anticraving and antiwithdrawal effects weighed against possible side effects. Maintenance bromocriptine treatment may be necessary if symptoms recur after discontinuation.

sents correction of cocaine-withdrawal-induced imbalances, spontaneous remission of stimulant withdrawal, or improvement in coexisting affective illness. Furthermore, tricyclic antidepressants produce some of the same neurochemical disruptions seen in cocaine administration, such as blockade of norepinephrine reuptake and increased postsynaptic dopamine sensitivity (Spyraki & Fibiger, 1981). Therefore, tricyclic antidepressants might conceivably aggravate cocaine-induced neurochemical imbalances in the norepinephrine and dopamine systems. In fact, relapses to cocaine have been reported after initiation of desipramine treatment (Weiss, 1989). Reported efficacy with desipramine could result from its ability to replace cocaine effects, rather than reverse imbalances.

CONCLUSIONS

This chapter has reviewed medical, neurochemical, and neuroendocrine disruptions caused by the acute and chronic administration of cocaine, with emphasis on clinical relevance. It should be obvious that significant alterations occur in the pleasure centers of the brain and that persistent abnormalities lead to withdrawal and craving states. Alterations in endogenous reward centers, when considered along with the intense euphoria of cocaine intoxication, unquestionably define this drug as "physically" addictive. Furthermore, in light of its medical complications, cocaine can be described as addictive and medically dangerous, in spite of dated mythology to the contrary. Besides contributing to our knowledge of endogenous reward centers, the neurochemical effects of cocaine point toward logical treatment interventions that can be researched and applied to this serious and expanding disorder. This application has been made in the form of bromocriptine for cocaine craving and withdrawal. Agents that restore balance in the serotonin, norepinephrine, thyroid, and other systems may also prove to have important roles in the management of cocaine patients. Other pharmacological interventions are needed to reverse cocaine overdose, the progression of the addiction, cocaine-induced depression, and cocaine euphoria. When used in conjunction with effective rehabilitation, new pharmacological treatments should enhance recovery rates of patients treated for cocaine abuse.

REFERENCES

Areosty, D. J., Stanley, R. B., Jr. & Crockett, D. M. (1986) Pneumomediastinum and cervical emphysema from the inhalation of "freebase" cocaine: Report of three cases. *Head Neck Surg.* 94:372–374.

Barth, C. W., Bray, M. & Roberts, W. C. (1986) Rupture of the ascending aorta during cocaine intoxication. *Am. J. Cardiol.* 57:496.

Bates, C. K. (1988) Medical risks of cocaine use. *West. J. Med.* 148:440–444.

Berger, P., Gawin, F. & Kosten, T. R. (1989) Treatment of cocaine abuse with mazindol. *Lancet* i:283.

Bingol, H., Fuchs, M., Diaz, V., Stone, R. K. & Gromish, D. S. (1987) Teratogenicity of cocaine in humans. *J. Pediat.* 110:93–96.

Bozarth, M. A. & Wise, R. A. (1985) Toxicity associated with long-term intravenous heroin and cocaine self-administration in the rat. *JAMA* 254:81-83.

Chaisson, R. E., Bacchetti, P., Osmond, D., Brodie, B., Sande, M. A. & Moss, A. R. (1989) Cocaine use and HIV infection in intravenous drug users in San Francisco. *JAMA* 261:561–565.

Chasnoff, I. J., Burns, W. J., Schnoll, S. H. & Burns, K. A. (1985) Cocaine use in pregnancy. *N. Engl. J. Med.* 313:666–669.

Chasnoff, I. J., Busseyne, A. B., Savich, R. & Stack, C. M. (1986) Perinatal cerebral infarction in maternal cocaine use. *J. Pediat.* 108:456–459.

Chasnoff, I. J., Griffith, D. R., MacGregor, S., Dirkes, K. & Burns, K. A. (1989) Temporal patterns of cocaine use in pregnancy. *JAMA* 261: 1741–1744.

Checkley, S. A. (1978) Corticosteroid and growth hormone responses to methyl-amphetamine in depressive illness. *Psychol. Med.* 8:1–9.

Cocores, J. A., Dackis, C. A. & Gold, M. S. (1986) Sexual dysfunction secondary to cocaine abuse in two patients. *J. Clin. Psychiat.* 47:384–385.

Corbett, D. & Wise, R. A. (1980) Intracranial self-stimulation in relation to the ascending dopaminergic systems of the midbrain: A moveable electrode mapping study. *Brain Res.* 185:1–15.

Cregler, L. L. & Mark, H. (1986) Medical complications of cocaine abuse. *N. Engl. J. Med.* 315:1495–1500.

Cregler, L. L. & Mark, H. (1987) Relation of stroke to cocaine abuse. *NY State J. Med.* 87:124–129.

Dackis, C. A., Estroff, T. W. & Gold, M. S. (1985) Hyperprolactinemia in cocaine abuse. *Am. Psych. Assoc. Abstr.* NR 181.

Dackis, C. A., Estroff, T. W., Sweeney, D. R., Pottash, A. L. C. & Gold, M. S. (1985a) Specificity of the TRH test for major depression in patients with serious cocaine abuse. *Am. J. Psychiat.* 142:1097–1099.

Dackis, C. A., Estroff, T. W., Sweeney, D. R., Pottash, A.L.C. & Gold, M. S. (1985b) Thyroid axis abnormalities in cocaine abuse. *National Institute of Drug Abuse, Research Monograph Series* 55:254–257.

Dackis, C. A. & Gold, M. S. (1985a) New concepts in cocaine addiction: The dopamine depletion hypothesis. *Neurosci. Biobev. Rev.* 9:469–477.

Dackis, C. A. & Gold, M. S. (1985b) Bromocriptine as a treatment of cocaine abuse. *Lancet* 1:1151–1152.

Dackis, C. A. & Gold, M. S. (1985c) Pharmacological approaches to cocaine addiction. *J. Subst. Abuse Treatment* 2: 139–145.

Dackis, C. A. & Gold, M. S. (1987) Substance-induced psychiatric disorders. *Am. Psych. Assoc. Symposium Abstracts.*

Dackis, C. A., Gold, M. S., Annitto, W. J. & Davies, R. K. (1986) Bromocriptine reverses post-cocaine depression. *Soc. Neurosci. Abstr.* 12:477.

Dackis, C. A., Gold, M. S., Davies, R. K. & Sweeney, D. R. (1985) Bromocriptine treatment for cocaine abuse: The dopamine depletion hypothesis. *Int. J. Psychiat. Med.* 15:125–135.

Dackis, C. A., Gold, M. S., Estroff, T. W. & Sweeney, D. R. (1984) Hyperprolactinemia in cocaine abuse. *Soc. Neurosci. Abstr.* 10:1099.

Dackis, C. A., Gold, M. S., Sweeney, D. R., Byron, J. P. & Climko, R. (1987) Single-dose bromocriptine reverses cocaine craving. *Psychiat. Res.* 20:261–264.

DiGiulio, A. M., Gropetti, A., Cattabeni, F., Galli, C. L., Maggi, A., Algeri, S. & Ponzio, F. (1971) Significance of dopamine metabolites in the evaluation of drugs acting on dopamine neurons. *Eur. J. Pharmacol.* 52:201–207.

Dimijian, G. G. (1974) Contemporary drug abuse. In: Goth, A. (Ed.), *Medical pharmacology* (7th ed.). St. Louis: C. V. Mosby, 313.

Dow Edwards, D. L. (1988) Developmental effects of cocaine. In: Clovet, D., Asghar, K. & Brow, R. (Eds.), *Mechanisms of cocaine abuse and toxicty.* NIDA Research Monograph 88. Washington, D.C.: Government Printing Office, 290–303.

Duke, M. (1986) Cocaine myocardial infarction and arrhythmias: A review. *Conn. Med.* 50:440–442.

Edvenson, R. & MacKinzie, P. (1976) Amine mechanisms in the cerebral circulation. *Pharmacol. Rev.* 28:275–348.

Extein, I. L., Gross, D. A. & Gold, M. S. (1986) Cocaine detoxification using bromocriptine. *Am. Psych. Assoc. Abstr.* (New Research Abstract # 70).

Extein, I., Potter, W. Z., Gold, M. S., Andre, P., Rafuls, W. A. & Gross, D. A. (1987) Persistent neurochemical deficit in cocaine abuse. *Am. Psych. Assoc. Abstr.* NR 61.

Gawin, F. H. & Ellinwood, E. (1988) Cocaine and other stimulants. *N. Engl. J. Med.* 318:1173–1182.

Gawin, F. H. & Kleber, H. D. (1984) Cocaine abuse treatment: Open pilot trial with desipramine and lithium carbonate. *Arch. Gen. Psychiat.* 41:903–909.

Gawin, F. H. & Kleber, H. D. (1985) Neuroendocrine findings in chronic cocaine abusers: A preliminary report. *Br. J. Psychiat.* 147:569–573.

Gawin, F. H. & Kleber, H. D. (1986) Abstinence symptomatology and psychiatric diagnosis in cocaine abusers. *Arch. Gen. Psychiat.* 43:107–113.

Geggel, R. L., McInerny, J. & Estes, N. (1989) Transient neonatal ventricular tachycardia associated with maternal cocaine use. *Am. J. Cardiol.* 63:383–384.

Goeders, N. E. & Smith, J. E. (1983) Cortical dopaminergic involvement in cocaine reinforcement. *Science* 221:773–775.

Gold, M. S., Pottash, A.L.C. & Extein, I. (1982) "Symptomless" autoimmune thyroiditis in depression. *Psychiat. Res.* 6:261–269.

Gold, M. S., Redmond, D. E. & Kleber, H. D. (1978) Clonidine in opiate withdrawal. *Lancet* i(8070):929–930.

Gold, M. S., Washton, A. M. & Dackis, C. A. (1985) Cocaine abuse: Neuro-chemistry, phenomenology, and treatment. In: Kozel, N.J. & Adams, E. H. (Eds.), *Cocaine use in America: Ep-*

idemiologic and clinical perspectives. NIDA Research Monograph 61. Washington, D.C.: Government Printing Office, 130–150.

Howard, R. E., Heuter, D. C. & Davis, G. J. (1985) Acute myocardial infarction following cocaine abuse in a young woman with normal coronary arteries. *JAMA* 254:95–96.

Hueter, D. C. (1989) Cardiovascular effects of cocaine. *JAMA* 257:979–980.

Hurd, Y. L. & Ungerstedt, V. (1989) An in vivo microdialysis evaluation of its acute action on dopamine transmission in rat striatum. *Synapse* 3:48–54.

Isner, J. M., Estes, N.A.M., Thompson, P. D., Costanzo-Nordin, M. R., Subramanian, R., Miller, G., et al. (1986) Acute cardiac events temporarily related to cocaine abuse. *N. Engl. J. Med.* 315:1438–1443.

Itkonen, J., Schnoll, S. & Glassroth, J. (1984) Pulmonary dysfunction in "freebase" cocaine users. *Arch. Intern. Med.* 144:2195–2197.

Jaffe, J. (1987) Bromocriptine attenuates cocaine craving. Personal correspondence.

Jatlow, P. L. (1987) Drug of abuse profile: Cocaine. *Clin. Chem.* 33:66B–71B.

Jones, M. T., Millhouse, E. & Burden, J. (1976) Secretion of corticotropin-releasing hormone in vitro. In: Martini, L. & Ganong, W. F. (Eds.), *Frontiers in neuroendocrinology*. New York: Raven Press, 195–226.

Jonsson, S., O'Meara, M. & Young, J. B. (1983) Acute cocaine poisoning: Importance of treating seizures and acidosis. *Am. J. Med.* 75:1061–1064.

Khaye, B. & Fainstadt, M. (1987) Cerebral vasculitis associated with cocaine use. *JAMA* 258:2104–2106.

Kirkby, R. J. & Petchkovsky, L. (1973) Chronic administration of cocaine: Effects on defecation and adrenal hypertrophy in the rat. *Neuropharmacology* 12:101.

Langner, N. O., Bement, C. L. & Perry, L. E. (1988) Arteriosclerotic toxicity of cocaine. In: Clovet, D., Asghar, K. & Brow, R. (Eds.), *Mechanisms of cocaine abuse and toxicity*. NIDA Research Monograph 88. Washington, D.C.: Government Printing Office, 325–336.

MacFarland, J. E., Krauss, J. R., Hepler, R. S. & Shorr, N. (1989) Orbital inflamation and optic neuropathies associated with sinusitis from intranasal cocaine abuse. *Arch. Opht.* 107:831–835.

MacGregor, S. N., Keith, L. G., Chasnoff, I. J., Rosner, M. A., Chisum, G. M., Shaw, P. & Minoque, D. P. (1987) Cocaine use during pregnancy: Adverse perinatal outcome. *Am. J. Obstet. Gynecol.* 157:686–690.

MacLeod, R. M. (1976) Regulation of prolactin secretion. In: Martini, L. & Ganong, W. F. (Eds.), *Frontiers in neuroendocrinology*. New York: Raven Press, 169–194.

Mantegazza, P., Naimzada, K. M. & Riva, M. (1968) Activity of amphetamine in hypothyroid rats. *Eur. J. Pharmacol.* 5:10–16.

Meltzer, H. Y., Wiita, B., Tricou, B. J., et al. (1982) Effect of serotonin precursors and serotonin agonists on plasma hormone levels. *Adv. Biochem. Psychopharmacol.* 34:117–140.

Mendelson, J. H., Teoh, S. K., Lange, U., Mello, N., Weiss, R., Skupny, A. & Ellingboe, J. (1988). Anterior pituitary, adrenal, and gonadal hormones during cocaine withdrawal. *Am. J. Psychiat.* 145:1094–1098.

Moore, T., Sorg, J., Miller, L., Kety, E. & Resnick, R. (1986) The more dynamic effects of intravenous cocaine on the pregnant ewe and fetus. *Am. J. Obstet. Gynecol.* 155:883–888.

Morley, J. E., Shafer, R. B., Elson, M. K., Slag, M. F., Raleigh, M. J., Brammer, G. L., et al. (1980) Amphetamine-induced hyperthyroxinema. *Ann. Intern. Med.* 93:707.

Myers, J. A. & Earnest, M. P. (1984) Generalized seizures and cocaine abuse. *Neurology* 34:675–676.

Nahas, G., Trouve, R., Demus, J. F. & Von Sitbon, M. (1985) A calcium-channel blocker as antidote to the cardiac effects of cocaine intoxication. *N. Engl. J. Med.* 313:519–520.

Nakamura, G. R. & Nogvch, T. T. (1981) Fatalities from cocaine overdoses in Los Angeles County. *Clin. Toxicol.* 18:895–905.

Nolte, B. & Gelman, B. B. (1989) Intracerebral hemorrhage associated with cocaine abuse. *Arch. Pathol. Lab. Med.* 113:812–813.

O'Brien, P. Ch., Childness, A. R. & Arndt, I. O. (1988) Pharmacological and behavioral treatments of cocaine dependence. *J. Clin. Psychiat.* 49:17–22.

Patrick, R. L. & Barchas, J. D. (1977) Potentiation by cocaine of the stimulus-induced increase in dopamine synthesis in rat brain striatal synaptosomes. *Neuropharmacology* 16:327.

Post, R. M. (1975) Cocaine psychosis: A continuum model. *Am. J. Psychiat.* 132:225–231.

Post, R. M. (1981) Central stimulants. In: Yedy, I., Glaser, F. B. & Schmidt, W., et al. (Eds), *Research advances in alcohol and drug problems.* New York: Plenum Press, p. 6.

Post, R. M., Kopanda, R. T. & Black, K. E. (1976) Progressive effects of cocaine on behavior and central amine metabolism in the rhesus monkey:

Relationship to kindling and psychosis. *Biol. Psychiat.* 11:403–419.

Raff, M. (1976) Self-regulation of membrane receptors. *Nature* 259:265–266.

Rees, L. Butler, P.W.P. & Gosling, C. (1970) Adrenergic blockade and the corticosteroid and growth hormone responses to methylamphetamine. *Nature* 228:565.

Reichlin, S. (1975) Regulation of the hypophysiotropic secretions of the brain. *Arch. Intern. Med.* 135:1350–1361.

Resnick, R. P., Kestenbaum, R. S. & Schwartz, L. K. (1977) *Science* 195:696–698.

Ring, M. E. & Butman, S. M. (1986) Cocaine and premature myocardial infarction. *Drug Ther.* 16:117–125.

Ross, S. B. & Renyi, A. L. (1966) Uptake of some tritiated sympathomimetic amines by mouse brain cortex in vitro. *Acta. Pharmacol. Toxicol.* 24:297–309.

Rowbotham, M., et al. (1987) Neurologic and psychiatric complications associated with cocaine abuse. *Am. J. Med.* 83:841–846.

Saberi, M. & Utinger, R. D. (1983) Augmentation of thyrotropin response to thyrotropin-releasing hormone following small decreases in serum thyroid hormone concentrations. *J. Clin. Endocrinol. Metab.* 40:1145–1149.

Sachar, E. J., Asnis, G. & Nathan, S. (1980) Dextroamphetamine and cortisol in depression: Morning plasma cortisol levels suppressed. *Arch. Gen. Psychiat.* 37:755–757.

Salanova, V. & Taubner, R. (1984) Intracerebral hemorrhage and vasculitis secondary to amphetamine use. *Postgrad. Med. J.* 60:429–430.

Satel, S. & Gawin, F. H. (1989) Migraine-like headache and cocaine use. *JAMA* 261:2995–2996.

Schuster, Ch. R. (1987) The United States drug abuse scene: An overview. *Clin. Chem.* 33:7B–12B.

Schwartz, K. A. & Cohen, J. A. (1984) Subarachnoid hemorrhage precipitated by cocaine snorting. *Arch. Neurol.* 41:705.

Schweitzer, V. G. (1986) Osteolytic sinusitis and pneumomediastinum: Deceptive otolaryngologic complications of cocaine abuse. *Laryngoscope* 96:206–210.

Shannon, M. (1988) Clinical toxicity of cocaine adulterants. *Ann. Emerg. Med.* 17:1243–1247.

Sherer, D. A., Kumor, K. A., Cone, E. J. & Jaffe, J. H. (1988) Suspiciousness induced by four-hours intravenous infusion of cocaine. *Arch. Gen. Psychiat.* 45:673–677.

Siegel, R. K. (1978) Cocaine hallucinations., *Am. J. Psychiat.* 135:309–314.

Siegel, R. K. (1982) Cocaine and sexual dysfunction: The curse of mama coca. *J. Psychoactive Drugs* 14:71.

Simpson, R. W. & Edwards, W. D. (1986) Pathogenesis of cocaine-induced ischemic heart disease. *Arch. Pathol. Lab. Med.* 110:479–484.

Smith, R. F., Muttran, K. M. & Kurkjian, M. F. (1989) Alterations in offspring behavior induced by chronic prenatal cocaine dosing. *Neurotoxicol. and Teratol.* 11:33–38.

Spear, L. P., Kirstein, C., Bell, J., Greenbaum, R., O'Shea, J., Tootianasumpun, V., et al. (1987) Effects of prenatal cocaine on behavior during the early postnatal period in rats. *Teratology* 35:BTS12.

Spyraki, C. & Fibiger, H. C. (1981) Behavioral evidence for supersensitivity of postsynaptic dopamine receptors in the mesolimbic system after chronic administration of desipramine. *Eur. J. Pharmacol.* 74:195–206.

Stevens, J. R., Mark, V. H., Irwin, S., Pacheco, E. & Suematzo, K. (1969) The temporal stimulation in man, long latency, long-lasting psychological changes. *Arch. Neurol.* 21:157–169.

Tashkin, D. P., Simmons, M. S., Coulson, A. H., Clark, V. A. & Gong, H., Jr. (1987) Respiratory effects of cocaine freebasing among habitual users of marijuana with or without tobacco. *Chest* 92:638–644.

Taylor, D., Ho, B. T. & Fagen, J. D. (1979) Increased dopamine receptor binding in rat brain by repeated cocaine injections. *Commun. Psychopharmacol.* 3:137–142.

Tennant, F. S. (1985) Effect of cocaine dependence on plasma phenylalanine and tyrosine levels and on urinary MHPG excretion. *Am. J. Psychiat.* 142:1200–1201.

Tennant, F. S. (Ed.) (1986) *Medical withdrawal from cocaine dependence with amantadine and other Parkinsonian drugs.* West Covina, Calif.: Veract, 7.

Tennant, F. S. & Sagherian, A. A. (1987) Double-blind comparison of amantadine hydrochloride and bromocriptine mesylate for ambulatory withdrawal from cocaine dependence. *Arch. Intern. Med.* 147:109–112.

Togna, G., Tempesta, E. & Togna, A. R. (1985) Platelet responsiveness and biosynthesis of thromboxane and protocyclin in response to in vitro cocaine treatment. *Haemostasis* 15:100–107.

Trulson, M. T. & Ulissey, M. J. (1986) Chronic cocaine administration decreases dopamine synthesis rates and increases ^3H spiroperidol binding in rat brain. *Brain Res. Bull.* 19:35–38.

Van Dyke, C. & Byck, R. (1977) Cocaine in 1884–1974. In: Ellinwood, E. (Ed.), *Advances in behavioral biology.* Plenum Press, 1–30.

Van Dyke, C. & Byck, R. (1982) Cocaine. *Sci. Am.* 246:128–141.

Vilensky, W. (1982) Illicit and licit drugs causing perforation of the nasal septum. *Forensic Sci.* 313:666–669.

Volkow, N. D., Mullani, N., Gould, L. K., Adler, S. & Krajewski, K. (1988) Cerebral blood flow in chronic cocaine users. *British J. Psychiatry* 152:641–648.

Walla, M. B. & Gershon, S. (1971) A neuropsychopharmacological comparison of D-amphetamine, L-DOPA and cocaine. *Neuropharmacology* 10:743–752.

Washton, A. M. & Gold, M. S. (1984) Chronic cocaine abuse: Evidence for adverse effects on health and functioning. *Psych. Annals* 14:733–743.

Weingarten, K. (1988) Cerebral vasculitis associated with cocaine abuse as subarachnoid hemorrhage. *JAMA* 259:1648–1649.

Weiss, R. D. (1989) Relapse to cocaine abuse after initiating desipramine treatment. *JAMA* 260:2545–2546.

Weiss, R. D., Goldenheim, P. D., Mirin, S. M., Hales, C. A. & Mendelson, J. H. (1981) Pulmonary dysfunction in cocaine smokers. *Am. J. Psychiat.* 138:1110–1112.

Wetli, C. V. (1981) Investigation of drug-related deaths: An overview. *Am. J. Forensic Sci.* 26:492–500.

Wilkerson, D. R. (1988) Cardiovascular toxicity of cocaine. In: Clovet, D., Asghar, K. & Brow, R. (Eds.) *Mechanisms of cocaine abuse and toxicity.* NIDA Research Monograph 88. Washington, D.C.: Government Printing Office, 304–325.

Wise, R. A. (1984) Neural mechanisms of the reinforcing action of cocaine. In: Grabowski, J. (Ed.), *Cocaine: Pharmacology, effects, and treatment of abuse.* NIDA Research Monograph 50, DHHS pub. no. (ADM) 84-1326. Washington, D.C.: Government Printing Office, 15–33.

Wise, R. A., Spindler, J., de Wit, H. & Gerber, G. J. (1978) Neuroleptic-induced "anhedonia" in rats: Pimozide blocks the reward quality of food. *Science* 201:262–264.

Wojak, J. C. & Flamm, E. S. (1987) Intracranial hemorrhage and cocaine use. *Stroke* 18:712–713.

Woods, J. R., Plessinger, M. A. & Clark, K. E. (1987) Effects of cocaine on uterine blood flow and fetal oxygenation. *JAMA* 257:957–961.

8

Consequences and Correlates of Cocaine Abuse: Clinical Phenomenology

Frank H. Gawin and Everett H. Ellinwood, Jr.

This chapter describes clinical consequences of cocaine abuse as well as the limits of extant knowledge. Many elements contribute to the presentations currently seen clinically, including: recent cultural changes and older historical forces, acute stimulant euphoria and acute postuse dysphoria, the route of administration, neurochemical effects, medical consequences, the phase of transition to dependence, abstinence phases and symptoms, and interactions with psychiatric disorder. All of these require understanding before the clinical presentation of any cocaine abuser can be adequately interpreted. Consequently, this chapter briefly reviews pertinent history and epidemiology, acute stimulant effects, and medical morbidity to provide a foundation for the discussion of clinical psychiatric presentations.

ACUTE ACTIONS

Cocaine, amphetamine, and similar stimulants are self-administered in pursuit of intensified pleasure. Acutely, these stimulants produce profound subjective well-being with alertness. Normal pleasures are magnified. Anxiety is decreased. Self-confidence and self-perceptions of mastery increase. Social inhibitions are reduced and interpersonal communication is facilitated. All aspects of the personal environment take on intensified qualities, but without hallucinatory perceptual distortions. Emotionality and sexual feelings are enhanced (Freud, 1884; Lasagna et al., 1955; Lewin, 1924; Nathanson, 1937; Van Dyke et al., 1982).

While stimulant use is initially enjoyable and seemingly easily controlled, repeated use gradually produces obsessions over recapturing stimulant-induced euphoria and extreme, compulsive urges for more use. This alters behavior and often causes severe psychological distress.

Stimulants with high abuse potential activate mesolimbic and or mesocortical dopaminergic pathways to produce euphoria (Goeders & Smith, 1983; Yokel & Wise, 1983). In animals electrical self-stimulation of these pathways mirrors stimulant self-administration. Increases in behavioral and physiological reward indices are produced by either electrical stimulation of these dopaminergic reward regions or by stimulants. Such increases in reward are decreased by pharmacological dopamine receptor blockade or lesions in dopaminergic reward pathways. The neurochemical and neuroanatomical localization of stimulant euphorigenic effects in dopaminergic reward regions is extremely important because it provides new avenues toward understanding and researching both stimulant withdrawal and potential treatments.

CLINICAL CHARACTERISTICS AND TREATMENT

Many consistent clinical reports on the characteristics of cocaine and amphetamine abusers appearing for treatment exist in the literature. Observations from the beginning of this century (Lewin, 1924; Maier, 1926), through the latest United States amphetamine epidemic of 1967–1972 (Connell, 1970; Ellinwood, 1967; Kramer et al., 1967; Smith, 1969), and the current surge in cocaine abuse (Gawin & Kleber, 1986a; Gold et al., 1985; Siegel, 1982) all indicate (1) that predictable psychiatric complications can occur acutely during or after individual episodes or "binges" of stimulant abuse and (2) that chronic abuse can be associated with separate chronic psychiatric sequelae, particularly mood dysfunctions. Clinical presentations often include a mixture of acute and chronic symptoms with differing intensities of each. Separation of these dimensions requires ongoing longitudinal assessments.

ACUTE COCAINE-USE SEQUELAE

Cocaine Intoxication

Cocaine euphoria is phenomenologically distinct from opiate, alcohol, or other substance-induced euphorias. As noted earlier, qualities of acute intoxication in usual street dosages include euphoria, activation, decreased anxiety (initially), disinhibition, heightened curiosity and increased interest in the personal environment, feelings of increased competence and self-esteem, and a clear sensorium without hallucinations or cognitive confusion. Adverse consequences can result from atypical reactions or exaggerations of these sought-after components of the cocaine "high." Exaggerations include extreme euphoric disinhibition, impaired judgment, grandiosity, impulsiveness, irresponsibility, atypical generosity, hypersexuality, hypervigilance, compulsive repetitive actions, and extreme psychomotor activation. Adverse sequelae include the psychosocial and economic consequences of actions undertaken while intoxicated, such as abrogation of responsibilities, loss of money, sexual indiscretions, or atypical illegal activities, but can also include physical injury that results from dangerous acts performed while judgment is impaired.

Complications such as acute psychiatric disorders or medical emergencies may occur. Marked cocaine intoxication strongly resembles the mania or hypomania of bipolar psychiatric disorder, and can sometimes trigger mania. If cocaine activation is not self-remitting within less than 24 hours in an observed, cocaine-free setting, then mania is probably present.

Cocaine Delirium

Euphoric stimulation can become dysphoric as the dosage and duration of administration increase. In most cocaine binges, an admixture of anxiety and irritability soon accompany the desired euphoric effects. Anxiety ranges from mild dysphoric stimulation to extreme paranoia or a panic-like delirium. In moderate form, a state of global sympathetic discharge occurs, which strongly resembles a panic anxiety attack, and is often associated with fear of impending death from cocaine. Disorientation is not usually present, except in very severe cases.

Cocaine Delusions

Delusional psychoses occur after prolonged and intense cocaine binges. These have also been experimentally induced by amphetamine in unselected normals, and appear related to the amount and duration of stimulant administration rather than to predisposition to psychosis (Bell, 1970). Identical experiments have not been done with cocaine, but the clinical reports are similar. The delusional content is usually paranoid, and if it is mild, the stimulant abuser may retain awareness that induced fears are a consequence of the immediately preceding stimulant intake (Ellinwood, 1967). If severe, however, reality testing is completely impaired and caution is required. Case reports exist of homicides based in delusional self-defense against imagined threats (Ellinwood & Petrie, 1977).

Cocaine delusions are usually transient and remit within 24 hours of sleep normalization. Longer episodes, however, have been described after very prolonged binges, or in individuals having preexistent schizophrenic or manic psychoses. Short-term neuroleptic treatment is routinely used to ameliorate delusional symptomatology. Cocaine psychoses are considered to be due to dopaminergic activation, and the paradox of how activation of the dopaminergic system can produce such disparate states as paranoia and euphoria may hold important clues to understanding their CNS substrates (Gawin, 1986b). Flash-back phenomena or delayed reemergence of symptoms have not been described for stimulant-induced psychoses.

Postcocaine Dysphoria

If a stimulant-use episode involves several serial readministrations and/or substantial doses (a binge), even in a naive, nondependent user, then mood does not return to baseline when use ceases but instead rapidly descends into dysphoria. This dysphoria, called the "crash" by abusers, is usually self-limited, resolving after one or two nights of sleep. Clinically, the crash fully mimics unipolar depression with melancholia, except for its comparatively brief duration. It is a regular accompaniment of the recurrent binges that occur in cocaine dependence, and is discussed more fully in a later section on chronic cocaine dependence.

The depression of the crash can be extremely intense, and may include potentially lethal, but temporary, suicidal ideation, which remits completely when the crash is over. This transient suicidal ideation can occur in individuals who have no prior history of depression, suicidal ideation, or suicide attempts. True unipolar depression (which is not self-remitting and requires antidepressant treatment) may also occur, but only in a reduced subpopulation, as discussed later in this chapter. Clinical management includes, first, observation to prevent self-harm while providing an opportunity for sleep and recovery of mood, and second, evaluation after sleep to ensure that neurovegetative symptoms and suicidal ideation have remitted.

CHRONIC COCAINE ABUSE

Constraints on Knowledge

Although the full extent of morbidity caused by chronic stimulant abuse is unknown, many different types of adverse consequences have been identified, ranging from medical complications (including overdose, pathology due to administration route, neurotoxicity), to psychiatric disorders, to psychosocial disruption without clear physiological or psychiatric insult. Preclinical and clinical assessment of stimulant abuse have been far from exhaustive. Surprisingly, there are no human data that rigorously define the chronic medical or psychiatric consequences of long-term cocaine or amphetamine abuse, and few animal studies have been designed to reflect chronic human abuse. Most of what is known is based on survey data such as Drug Abuse Warning Network (DAWN) emergency room reports (or telephone surveys with inherent limitations based on sample self-selection), on clinical observations of single cases or small samples, or on animal data with questionable generalizability. Such research helps define the range, or types, of confirmed or suspected adverse cocaine sequelae but does not specify the extent, or quantity, of the sequelae, nor their likelihood for a given abuser. The available data therefore provide only a starting point for understanding the chronic clinical consequences of cocaine abuse.

Further, few systematic, large-scale clinical investigations of either the clinical psychiatric consequences of stimulant abuse, or their treatment, exist. We have only recently witnessed the appearance of systematic observations of abuse and abstinence patterns, of well-designed treatment experiments, and of refined conceptualizations of stimulant abuse and dependence. Rigorous substantiation is needed in all areas. Much of the following discussion is therefore based on clinical consensus, rather than on the precise, scientific observation or experimentation available for some other psychiatric and substance abuse disorders.

Early Cocaine Use

Cocaine use occurs across a wide spectrum. Despite the impressions produced by publicity on adverse effects, the majority of human stimulant use may be relatively benign. In the early 1960s millions of individuals were prescribed chronic amphetamines for depression or weight loss. Millions of amphetamine abusers clearly did not develop. Most patients were successfully, and relatively easily, weaned from stimulants when restrictions were applied because use had become uncontrolled in small subgroups. Similarly, the National Institute on Drug Abuse estimated that in 1985, of 30 million persons who had tried cocaine in the United States, only 6 million were regular users, and only one-fourth of those were in immediate need of treatment. Ninety five percent of those who had tried cocaine were therefore not apparently impaired. These data indicate that some individuals use cocaine intermittently, and that even low-intensity regular use can be controlled or successfully discontinued, as occurred with amphetamine in the preceding stimulant epidemic.

Development of cocaine dependence takes place within a social/occupational matrix. Initially, low doses enhance interactions with the environment, facilitating performance and confidence to enable productive increases in interpersonal or occupational industry and adventurousness (Connell, 1970; Ellinwood & Petrie, 1977; Gawin & Kleber, 1985b; Siegel, 1985). Euphoria in early stimulant use thus primarily results from increasingly positive external feedback to the user, rather than from direct pharmacological effects; it is often misperceived by the user as originating in the environment rather than in the drug. Combined with absent or scarcely apparent negative contingencies, such early experiences are quite seductive (Ellinwood & Petrie, 1977; Kleber & Gawin, 1984).

What distinguishes those who can easily cease stimulant use and do not progress beyond the experience just described from those who cannot, and how can the capacity to cease use be restored? With the exception of one study of recreational cocaine users by Siegel (1985), no detailed data on controlled cocaine users exist. Telephone "hot-line" surveys provide little information on controlled use since these lack clinical detail. Further, caller characteristics (Gold et al., 1985) are similar to treatment samples, rather than to community survey populations. Detailed abuse reports are, however, available from patients who develop dyscontrol and appear for treatment; retrospective data from these abusers, combined with judicious applications of animal data, provide a preliminary answer to the questions posed.

The "High-Intensity Transition"

Animals given free access to cocaine in preclinical studies engage in continuous self-administration. Death from cardiorespiratory collapse or infection follows within days (reviewed in Johanson, 1984). Cocaine and amphetamine are chosen over food, sex, opiates, alcohol, sedatives, hallucinogens, and phencyclidine. In limited administration paradigms, animals can be kept alive, but they generally adjust self-administration to maintain maximum effects within the limits of the paradigm (Groppetti et al., 1974). Human abusers who are severely impaired react similarly. They report virtual exclusion of all noncocaine-related thoughts during cocaine binges. Sex, nourishment, sleep, safety, survival, money, morality, loved one, and responsibility all become immaterial when juxtaposed with the desire to reexperience stimulant euphoria (Ellinwood & Petrie, 1977; Gawin & Kleber, 1986a; Lasagna et al., 1955; Lewin, 1924;

Siegel, 1982). Supplies of money or stimulants are drawn on until they are exhausted. Abuse is limited only by access, and human abusers appear to function like the nonhumans in preclinical studies.

Paradoxically, heavy human abusers report being similar to the millions of noncompulsive users during their early cocaine usage (Gawin & Kleber, 1985b). No animal studies report a similar low-intensity use. A phenomenon we term the "high-intensity transition" to compulsive use may underlie this paradox. Abusers report that compulsive use begins when the route of administration changes to one of rapid absorption (intravenous and smoking), or when drug availability and dosage increase markedly (e.g., increased resources, improved supply sources, engaging in cocaine commerce). Cocaine use is controlled, then, until episodes of extremely intense euphoria have occurred. Such episodes produce what become "persecutory memories" of the intense euphoria. These memories are later contrasted to any immediate dysphoria to become the fount of stimulant craving. Initially, high-intensity episodes are precluded by drug costs and availability and by concerns over safety that limit both the amounts used and any experimentation with rapid administration routes.

Consistent with this explanation, noncompulsive use has not been described for intravenous or smoking administration, which uniformly produces very intense euphoria (Kleber & Gawin, 1984; Siegel, 1982, 1985). Intranasal or oral administration routes produce intense euphoria if initial doses are large enough, but they are less likely to produce the transition because of slower absorption.

Chronic animal studies employ substantial cocaine boluses, often via intravenous administration. In effect, they begin at the high-intensity transition, which explains the lack of animal data on low-intensity use or the transition itself. Systematic clinical studies to examine the high-intensity transition, or any other explanation of the apparent dichotomy of stimulant use and abuse, have not been done. Both animal and clinical studies are clearly needed.

Popular misconception has held that intranasal cocaine use does not lead to abuse and that severe abuse requires daily administration. Both of these conceptions appear to be wrong. Treatment data from multiple sources show that more than 50% of cocaine abusers who seek treatment are exclusively intranasal users, with no differences in impairment between administration routes (reviewed in

Kleber & Gawin, 1984). Preliminary reports indicate that 90% of abusers appearing for treatment use cocaine in extended binges that disrupt sleep (Gawin & Kleber, 1985b), duplicating a pattern previously observed in amphetamine abusers (Connell, 1970; Kramer et al., 1967). Several days of abstinence often separate binges, and abusers report that limited daily use patterns precede binge abuse (Connell, 1970; Gawin & Kleber, 1985b). In contrast to nonstimulant substance abuse, daily stimulant use is to a maximal abuse pattern if normal sleep patterns are maintained, and severe abuse can exist without incessant daily administration. Rather than spreading out a cocaine purchase by using a few doses daily to make it last several weeks, as abusers do earlier in their histories, the established user exhausts all potentially available cocaine before terminating a binge. Some abusers with unlimited access do develop an unceasing binge lasting weeks or months with severely disrupted functioning (Siegel, 1982), but such cases are rare.

No personality predispositions to stimulant abuse have been demonstrated. However, major psychiatric mood and attention disorders, where stimulants are used as self-medication, are overrepresented in treatment (reviewed below). Genetic predisposition to stimulant abuse could exist; alcohol abuse in family members has been extensively commented upon by clinicians but has not been systematically studied. Nor have studies been done of genetic factors in stimulant-abusing populations. Taken together, the animal data and clinical data presently available clearly support only three clinically applicable predictors of cocaine abuse susceptibility or severity: use patterns (binges), availability (amount and administration route), and impairment of self-control (inability to ration supplies). More circumscribed categorizations of stimulant abuse are being proposed and evaluated, but are as yet arbitrary and inconclusive. These are discussed by the authors and others elsewhere (Gawin & Kleber, 1986a; Gold et al., 1985; Kleber & Gawin, 1984; Siegel, 1982, 1985).

Abstinence Phases

The existence and qualities of cocaine withdrawal are subjects of current controversy. This reflects dissimilarity between cocaine and opiates or alcohol. Classic pharmacological drug abuse constructs—such as withdrawal, dependence, and tolerance—do not provide models that can easily be applied to cocaine or other stimulants. Dependence and withdrawal, as measured by gross physiological indices, verge on being imperceptible in stimulant abusers. This accounts for the common perception that cocaine and amphetamine are only "psychologically" addictive. Reflecting the belief that cocaine abuse does not lead to dependence or withdrawal, the third edition of the *Diagnostic and Statistical Manual of Mental Disorders* (DSM-III) contained no diagnostic category for cocaine dependence. The revised manual, DSM-III(R); now contains this category for cocaine.

Chronic stimulant abuse regularly produces cyclical reoccurrences of use, as well as time-dependent evolution of abstinence symptoms. We have recently described a triphasic cocaine abstinence pattern that dispels the perception that cocaine use produces no withdrawal (see Gawin & Kleber, 1986a); this abstinence pattern is discussed in the following sections. We first describe all the stages of abstinence, accompanied by pertinent data from the animal literature, to account for an emerging conception of neurophysiologically based stimulant dependence. We then review special implications of the possible coexistence of DSM-III axis 1 psychiatric disorders.

Crash: Acute Dysphoria (Phase 1).

When euphoria decreases during a binge of stimulant use, anxiety, fatigue, irritability, and depression increase (see previous section on acute sequelae). This usually leads to stimulant readministration and prolonged binges. Supplies are eventually exhausted, however, or a state of extreme acute tolerance occurs in which further high-dose administration produces little euphoria; the anxiety of paranoia is augmented and self-administration ends. The "crash" is initially a descent into depressed mood with continued stimulation and anxiety. Then a desire for rest and escape from the hyperstimulated dysphoria develops. This often causes use of anxiolytics, sedatives, opiates, marijuana, or alcohol to induce sleep. Whether or not sleep is pharmacologically induced, hypersomnolence and hyperphagia (during brief awakenings or after the hypersomnolence) eventually occur. The duration of these periods is related to the duration and intensity of the preceding binge (Gawin & Kleber, 1986a).

Following week-long stimulant binges, hypersomnolence may last several days (Kramer et al., 1967; Siegel, 1982). Awaking from the hypersomnolence is usually associated with markedly improved mood, although some residual dysphoria may occur, particularly in high-intensity abusers. The exhaustion, depression, and hypersomnolence of the crash probably result from acute neurotransmitter depletion secondary to the preceding stimulant binge. Such depletion has been demonstrated directly in animal experiments (Taylor & Ho, 1977) and in experiments using indirect peripheral indices (Watson et al., 1972). Clinical recovery from the crash probably depends on sleep, diet, and time for new dopamine and norepinephrine synthesis. One report of precursor loading with tyrosine indicates that tyrosine decreases crash symptoms (Gold et al., 1983), but this report has not been replicated or extended to clinical treatment.

Clinical management of the crash was discussed earlier. The crash has sometimes been equated with a withdrawal state (Gold et al., 1983; Siegel, 1982; Smith, 1969). Acute tolerance to stimulant effects, occurring within a binge, has been clearly described clinically and in laboratory experiments (Fischman et al., 1976; Gawin & Kleber, 1985b). Furthermore, changes in peripheral catecholamine indices and sleep EEG immediately after stimulant administration have been used as support for the existence of a dependent state, at least for amphetamines (Watson et al., 1972). Unlike opiates and alcohol, however, stimulant abuse usually does not occur daily; chronic tolerance has not been experimentally proven and clinical consensus is that it is much less substantial; and craving is usually absent immediately after the crash and is only episodic later on (Connell, 1970; Gawin & Kleber, 1986a; Kramer et al., 1967; Siegel, 1982). In opiate or alcohol withdrawal, craving for the abused substance to alleviate withdrawal symptoms is rapid, marked, and continuous. Relapse directly follows such craving. Except in the beginning of the cocaine crash, however, craving occurs only for sleep or rest, and further stimulant use is often strongly rejected in the hope that sleep or rest may be attained (Gawin & Kleber, 1986a). It appears that the crash may be similar to immediate, high-dose alcohol aftereffects ("hangover"), rather than to alcohol or opiate withdrawal. The crash thus appears to be a *self-limiting acute* state that does not itself require active treatment. It apparently does not contribute to chronic relapse and abuse, but only to prolonged stimulant binges (Gawin & Kleber, 1986a).

Withdrawal: Poststimulant Mood Dysfunction (Phase 2).

The nervous system's usual response to persistent, drug-induced neurochemical perturbation is compensatory adaptation in the perturbed system. Dysregulation occurs when the drug is not present. Despite the recent perception that stimulants may only be "psychologically" addictive, it is illogical to assume that neuroadaptation does not occur in stimulant abuse. This does not mean a classic drug abstinence syndrome uniformly occurs; instead chronic, high-dose stimulant use could generate sustained neurophysiological changes in brain systems that regulate psychological processes only. Changes in these neurophysiological systems could produce a true physiological addiction and withdrawal, but one whose clinical expression is psychological.

Both extensive experimental data in animals and clinical evidence support this view. Briefly, animal experiments using electrical stimulation at brain reward sites that are activated by cocaine show a decrease in sensitivity after chronic stimulant administration (Colpaert et al., 1979; Kokkinidis & Zacharko, 1980; Leith & Barrett, 1976). This decrease is reversible with chronic antidepressant administration (Kokkinidis & Zacharko, 1980; Simpson, 1974). Human stimulant abusers display a symptom constellation, described below, that is consistent with a decreased capacity to perceive reward or pleasure. Further, chronic stimulants produce long-term animal neurotransmitter and neuroreceptor changes (Banerjee et al., 1979; Borison et al., 1979; Chanda et al., 1979; Ricuaurte et al., 1980; Taylor et al., 1979), animal behavioral changes (Utena, 1966; Yagi, 1963), and human neuroendocrine and sleep EEG changes (Gawin & Kleber, 1985a; Watson et al.; 1972). These all support the presence of a neuroadaptive process. These data are complex and are critically reviewed in more detail by Swann in this book.

Protracted dysphoria, occurring long after the crash, has been clinically identified in cocaine and amphetamine abusers (Connell, 1970; Gawin & Kleber, 1986a). Protracted dysphoric symptoms are frequent antecedents of stimulant craving, often leading to unceasing cycles of recurrent binges. These chronic symptoms are not quickly self-remitting and therefore have great importance in determining treatment. They thus have greater clinical similarity to "withdrawal" in other substances of abuse than do other abstinence symptoms such as the crash.

In most heavy cocaine abusers, a regular symptom progression follows the resolution of intoxication and crash symptoms. Upon awakening from hypersomnolence, a euthymic interval with normal mood and no stimulant craving occurs. In abusers attempting to cease use, the interval is usually associated with vivid memories of the misery of the crash and acute awareness of the psychosocial costs of continued abuse. This lasts from several hours to several days (Gawin & Kleber, 1986a). It is slowly supplanted by increasing inactivation, amotivation, and restricted pleasurable responses to the environment. These symptoms have been variously labeled anergia, depression (Connell, 1970; Kramer et al., 1967), anhedonia (Gawin & Kleber, 1984; Gawin & Kleber, 1986a), or psychasthenia (Ellinwood & Petrie, 1977) by different clinical observers.

The symptoms wax and wane; they are often not constant or severe enough to meet psychiatric diagnostic criteria for major affective disorders. The abuser's limited hedonic reactions to existence, contrasted with memories of cocaine-induced euphoria, nonetheless make resumption of use compellingly seductive. Furthermore, the symptom intensity is responsive to environmental cues—the same stimuli that trigger memories of cocaine euphoria and craving for cocaine also intensify awareness of an abuser's baseline dysphoria. During craving there appears to be a "state dependent" amplification of recall of cocaine euphoria and, simultaneously, a remarkable lack of memory for the crash or the adverse psychosocial consequences of abuse. Such negative memories often reemerge only when the episode of craving, and possibly relapse, has passed.

Anhedonic symptoms resolve within days to weeks of sustained abstinence (Connell, 1970; Ellinwood & Petrie, 1977; Gawin &

Kleber, 1986a; Smith, 1969). Animal studies in which sufficiently chronic and high-dose stimulants were administered report behavioral depression on withdrawal for a similar time period (Utena, 1966; Yagi, 1963). The severity and duration of these symptoms depend only partially on the intensity of the preceding chronic cocaine abuse. Predisposing mood disorders may also amplify these symptoms. Conversely, in intermittent, controlled stimulant users without psychiatric disorders, an anhedonic-psychasthenic phase may not occur at all. The high-intensity transition and coinciding neuroadaptation may be required before withdrawal psychasthenia and anhedonia emerge.

Extinction: Postwithdrawal Conditioned Dysfunction (Phase 3).

Following successful initiation of abstinence and the resolution of early anhedonia and craving, intermittent cocaine craving continues (Ellinwood & Petrie, 1977; Gawin & Kleber, 1986a; Maier, 1926). Such craving is not accompanied by the baseline dysphoria of the second phase, and potential neurophysiological mechanisms for these episodes are poorly understood. Cravings appear in the context of such divergent factors as particular mood states (positive as well as negative); specific persons, locations, events, or times of year; intoxications with other substances; interpersonal strife; or abuse objects (money, white powder, pipes, mirrors, syringes, single-edged razor blades, among many others). These factors vary; none are uniformly associated with craving. They appear to be conditioned cues, varying according to the abuse habits of the individual. Stimulants are the most potent reinforcing agents known (Johanson, 1984), and as such can be expected to produce classical and operant conditioning. Animal experiments have clearly established that strong conditioning to stimulants occurs. The craving is intense, and can reemerge months or even years after last stimulant use (Gawin & Kleber, 1986a). Conditioned craving is also reported during abstinence from other substances, although the authors' impression is that in former stimulant abusers conditioned cravings are more unpredictable and intense than in abusers of any other drugs.

No systematic studies of the reemergence of craving have been carried out, but clinical impressions indicate that such craving is episodic, lasting only hours with, in long-abstinent abusers, very long periods free of craving. The magnitude and episodisity of the craving, combined with the variety of the cues and their temporal contiguity to stimulant-abuse episodes, also support the view that this craving is classically conditioned.

The most common clinical example of a conditioned cue is alcohol. Alcohol disinhibition can overcome early hesitancies toward trying cocaine based on extreme expense or illegality. Thus, mild alcohol intoxication often precedes initial stimulant use or early repetitions of use. If this association occurs regularly, alcohol intoxication then becomes a conditioned cue for stimulant craving. Such abusers report little craving except immediately after alcohol intake. Relapse in such patients, often following successfully initiated abstinence, occurs with regularity when social contacts are reestablished after the weeks of relative social isolation imposed to facilitate early abstinence. Relapse occurs only after one or two drinks. In such cases individuals with years of nonproblematic recreational alcohol use, and total weekly alcohol intake of less than half a dozen drinks, may require total alcohol abstinence to become stimulant-free.

The conditioning hypothesis is testable and has important research and treatment implications. Systematic evaluations of conditioned craving and extinction techniques have recently begun, but reports are rare (Giannini, et al., 1986). Psychodynamic, behavioral, interpersonal, and psychosocial explanations for cocaine craving and relapse have all also been offered (Rounsaville et al., 1985; Wurmser, 1974). Contributions from each of these areas may exist, but have less immediate treatment relevance, and have limited scientific testability.

Chronic Stimulant-Induced Psychiatric Disorders

Do permanent neurotoxic changes occur as a consequence of cocaine abuse? Since most clinical and animal reports indicate that anhedonic symptoms decrease weeks to months after stimulant use ceases, clinical reports indicate that these changes are reversible. However, permanent dopaminergic neuronal degeneration has been documented in animal studies using amphetamines (Seiden, 1984) and is complemented by disturbing clinical observations. Reports from Scandinavia, Japan, and rare cases in the United States (Schuster & Fischman, 1985; Utena, 1966) describe chronic high-dose stimulant users, primarily intravenous amphetamine users, who have persistent anhedonia, anergia, and craving that do not remit, even after abstinence as long as 10 years. Preliminary investigations of whether the same neurotoxic changes occur in animals after cocaine have not been consistent, but cocaine's neurotoxicity may differ from that of amphetamine (Woolverton et al., 1987). Systematic long-term follow-up studies in abstinent former cocaine abusers are thus clearly needed.

Chronic amphetamine-induced paranoid psychoses have also been intermittently reported but in the context of how widespread stimulant abuse has been over the last two decades, they occur infrequently. It is not clear whether reported cases had preexistent psychiatric disorder, or whether cocaine is similar to amphetamine. Persistent cocaine-induced schizophreniform psychoses, induced by chronic rather than acute stimulant administration, have been expected on theoretical grounds (Post et al., 1976).

TREATMENT OF CHRONIC STIMULANT ABUSE

Most treatment for stimulant abuse in the United States consists of the same approaches as those used for alcohol or opiates, and it is applied without adaptation for specific problems associated with stimulant abuse (Kleber & Gawin, 1984). Specialized treatments are, however, being explored and developed. Interventions have sometimes been extreme, ranging from suggestions that treatment is unnecessary to the recent practice of bilateral cingulotomy in one South American country. Rational interventions have included adaptations of most major types of psychotherapy as well as pharmacotherapeutic trials (Anker & Crowley, 1982; Connell, 1970; Gawin & Kleber, 1984, 1986b; Gold et al., 1985; Khantzian & Khantzian, 1984; Kleber & Gawin, 1984; Maier, 1926; Rounsaville et al., 1985; Siegel, 1982; Wurmser, 1974). Pharmacotherapy trials make specific attempts to ameliorate clinical withdrawal symptomatology and hypothesized CNS changes due to cocaine, and are therefore summarized here.

Two observations have led to pharmacotherapy trials for cocaine withdrawal symptoms. First, changes in animal intracranial self-stimulation indices and neuroreceptor sensitivity after chronic treatment with tricyclic antidepressants are opposite to those demonstrated from chronic stimulants (Gawin & Kleber, 1984), and second, anecdotal reports show that antidepressants facilitate abstinence in psychasthenic-anhedonic amphetamine abusers (Ellinwood & Petrie, 1977). Open clinical trials of the tricyclic antidepressant, desipramine, produced abstinence in 92% of a group given desipramine compared with less than 50% in comparison groups given other agents (lithium and methylphenidate) or continued in psychotherapy without medication (Gawin & Kleber, 1984; Gawin, Riordan & Kleber, 1985). The trials were conducted primarily in nondepressed, psychotherapy-resistant, outpatient stimulant abusers to ensure that assessment occurred in severe abusers and that efficacy was not limited to abusers with major affective disorders. A simultaneous open trial with imipramine also demonstrated facilitated abstinence (Rosecan, 1983). Short-term tricyclic courses (Tennant, 1985), which are not associated with the neurophysiological changes of longer courses (Charney et al., 1981), did not facilitate abstinence. Although encouraging, these findings must be considered tentative; two larger-scale, double-blind, placebo-controlled studies have demonstrated the same trends (Gawin, Byck & Kleber, 1985; Giannini et al., 1986). Because antidepressants have not yet received FDA approval for the specific indication of cocaine withdrawal, they should not be routinely used clinically, except, of course, in stimulant abusers with concurrent affective disorder.

Other pharmacological treatment strategies have been proposed (Gawin & Kleber, 1984; 1986b; Gold et al., 1983; Jonsson et al., 1969; Rowbotham et al., 1984). Possible stimulant blockade has been tried using lithium, alpha-methylparatyrosine, trazodone, imipramine, or neuroleptics. These either have not demonstrated greater than partial blockade or have presented side effects that preclude compliance. Pilot attempts to increase dopaminergic neurotransmission using L-Dopa, tyrosine, amantadine, trihexylphenidyl, bromocriptine, and methylphenidate have reported short-term decreases in craving, but longer-term assessments are needed to assure that these effects are not transient (Dackis & Gold, 1985; Gawin, Riordan & Kleber, 1985; Gold et al., 1983; Khantzian, 1983;

Tennant, 1985). MAO inhibitors have also been reported to be useful in preventing relapse (Resnick & Resnick, 1984), but the potential dangers of using monoamine oxidase inhibitors (MAOI) and stimulants concurrently are unclear. Almost half the initial reports of death due to amphetamine involved MAOI interactions (Kalant & Kalant, 1979), and since it is not yet known if interactions with cocaine are less dangerous, trials with these agents have been limited. No systematic pharmacotherapy outcome trials were reported during the previous amphetamine epidemic.

It should be noted that experimental pharmacotherapies are being used to help initiate abstinence (though no long-term pharmacotherapy conferring enduring immunity to stimulant abuse is being tested in humans). Although some potential blocking agents have been tried clinically without evident blockade, and preclinical trials of new blocking agents are under way, there does not yet appear to be an agent to block relapse in cocaine abusers, as naltrexone does for opiate abusers.

DIAGNOSTIC CONSIDERATIONS

A presentation of stimulant use does not always indicate a diagnosis of cocaine abuse. The wide spectrum of cocaine use is reflected in the impression that a wider severity spectrum exists in cocaine abusers seeking treatment than in other substance abusers (Kleber & Gawin, 1984). Because of cocaine's now adverse reputation, its great expense, and the substantial amount of nonaddictive (or not-yet-addictive) use that exists, severe psychosocial disruption can lead to seeking treatment despite use in almost homeopathic amounts. When cocaine use is itself minor it may serve as a symptom of other primary problems, such as family discord, and alternative or adjunctive treatment may be indicated.

Coexistent psychiatric disorders appear frequently in cocaine-abuse treatment populations. Psychiatric patients can use cocaine as a misguided self-medication. Patients with major affective disorders, atypical depressive disorders, adult attention deficit disorder, bipolar or cyclothymic disorder, or narcolepsy have all been reported to cease illicit cocaine use when appropriate medications are substituted (Gawin & Kleber, 1984; Khantzian et al., 1984; Weiss et al., 1983). Schizophrenic patients have also been known to abuse amphetamines. Systematic studies using DSM-III criteria in cocaine abusers have found primary affective disorders to present in almost 50% of the stimulant abusers seeking treatment (Gawin, 1986a; Gawin & Kleber, 1985b; Weiss et al., 1983). Major depression appeared in approximately 10%–20% of cocaine abusers, dysthymic disorder in 10%–20%, and bipolar/cyclothymic disorder in 5%–15%. Acute aftereffects of a cocaine binge can mimic delusional or depressive disorders, and acute intoxication can mimic mania; it is therefore crucial to employ methods that separate out effects of acute stimulant use from enduring symptoms in clinical presentations. In the studies cited, this involved careful clinical interviewing during periods that were free of Phase 1 (crash) symptoms, about 9 to 14 days after last stimulant use, as well as searching personal histories for psychiatric symptoms during intervals free of substance abuse.

Since both substance abuse and psychiatric disorder often become evident in young adulthood, establishing a primary diagnosis in the manner described above is often difficult. Tentative diagnoses are therefore made based on symptom presentation, if several nights of sleep normalization and ensured abstinence (hospitalization or urinalysis) have occurred and depressive, manic, or psychotic symptoms have not remitted. Primary or secondary etiology can then be determined based on the subsequent clinical course, if abstinence is maintained. Sporadic stimulant use, however, often makes it possible to determine whether stimulant abuse or another axis 1 disorder is primary or secondary.

RESEARCH CONSIDERATIONS

Compared to, for example, affective disorders, both clinical and treatment data for stimulant abuse are at a primitive developmental stage. This chapter has summarized current knowledge. We would like to conclude, with the hope that more scientific cocaine-abuse treatment will evolve, by summarizing important methodological points for future cocaine-abuse research. The following points will all require clarification and consensus, through more definitive research, to achieve a coherent, scientifically acceptable body of data on cocaine abusers.

1. *Severity.* No studies reported thus far have stratified samples according to any criteria of abuse severity, and no generally accepted indices of severity of abuse exist that would allow comparisons across samples to be made.

2. *Self-selection artifacts.* Most clinical treatment or diagnostic studies have a substantial proportion of early dropouts or patients eliminated at screening who have not been contrasted to those remaining in treatment. Data characterizing the populations that find particular treatments aversive or inadequate are obviously needed, as are data on individuals who do not seek treatment.

3. *Recovery.* There is no consensus regarding how long abstinence must be maintained before recovery occurs or treatment can end. Outcome criteria are widely variable across the studies conducted thus far and, as of now, no studies have reported outcome in terms of changes in indices of psychosocial functioning.

4. *Heterogeneity.* Multiple sources of sample heterogeneity exist in cocaine treatment populations, including variations in sociodemographics, psychiatric symptomatology, psychosocial resources, patterns and duration of use, degree of impairment, treatment history, and other substances abused, among many others. Do such factors differ among treatment populations, and do they differentially affect clinical course or treatment outcome?

5. *Course and neuroadaptation.* There are few data available on the natural history of stimulant abuse, and few data available regarding which patients are likely to deteriorate, which may be expected to maintain stable states of dysfunction, and which will improve. This issue is related to the relative importance of preexisting psychopathology versus neuroadaptation. Although improved characterizations of abstinence symptoms have emerged, more systematic assessment, of clinical course are needed, and the contribution of neuroadaptation to continuation of human abuse requires further research and clarification.

ACKNOWLEDGMENTS

This chapter is an expanded and updated version of "Stimulant Dependence," Gawin, F. H. & Ellinwood, E. H., in Kleber, H. D. (Ed.), *Treatments of Psychiatric Disorders: A Task Force Report of the American Psychiatric Association.* Washington, D. C. : American Psychiatric Association, 1989.

The authors wish to thank Debra Gilbert, Joanne Firby, and Darlene Wyche-Alha-De for excellent editorial and secretarial assistance.

REFERENCES

Banerjee, S. P., Sharma, V. K., King-Cheung, L. S., Chanda, S. K. & Rigg, S. J. (1979) Cocaine and d-amphetamine induce changes in central β-adrenoceptor sensitivity: Effects of acute and chronic drug treatment. *Brain Res.* 175: 119–130.

Bell, D. S. (1970) The experimental reproduction of amphetamine psychosis. *Arch. Gen. Psychiat.* 127:1170–1175.

Borison, R. L., Hitri, A., Klawans, H. L. & Diamond, B. I. (1979) A new animal model for schizophrenia: Behavioral and receptor binding studies. In: Usdin, E. (Ed.), *Catecholamines: Basic and clinical frontiers.* New York: Pergamon Press.

Chanda, S. K., Sharma, W. K. & Banerjee, S. P. (1979) β-adrenoceptor sensitivity following psychotropic drug treatment. In: Usdin, E. (Ed.), *Catecholamines: Basic and clinical frontiers.* New York: Pergamon Press.

Charney, D. S., Menkes, D. B. & Heninger, G. R. (1981) Receptor sensitivity and the mechanism of action of antidepressant treatment. *Arch. Gen. Psychiat.* 38:1160–1180.

Colpaert, F. C., Niemegeers, C. J. & Janssen, P. A. (1979) Discriminative stimulus properties of cocaine: Neuropharmacological characteristics as derived from stimulus generalization experiments. *Pharmacol. Biochem. Behav.* 10: 535–546.

Connell, P. H. (1970) Some observations concerning amphetamine misuse: Its diagnosis, management, and treatment with special reference to research needs. In: Wittenborn, J. R., Brill, H. Smith, J. P. & Whittenborn, S. A. (Eds.), *Drugs and youth.* Springfield, Ill. : Charles C. Thomas.

Dackis, C. A. & Gold, M. S. (1985) Bromocriptine for cocaine withdrawal (Letter). *Lancet* 2:1151–1152.

Ellinwood, E. H. (1967) Amphetamine psychosis. I. Description of the individuals and process. *J. Nerv. Ment. Dis.* 144:273–283.

Ellinwood, E. H. & Petrie, W. M. (1977) Dependence on amphetamine, cocaine and other stimulants. In: Pradhan, S. N. (Ed.), *Drug abuse: Clinical and basic aspects.* New York: C. V. Mosby, 248–262.

Fischman, M. W., Schuster, C. R., Resnekiv, I., Schick, J. F. E., Krasnegor, N. A., Fannell, W. & Freedman, D. X. (1976) Cardiovascular and subjective effects of intravenous cocaine administration in humans. *Arch Gen. Psychiat.* 10: 535–546.

Freud, S. (1884) Uber Coca. *Zentbl. Ther.* 2:289–314.

Gawin, F. H. (1986a) Cocaine: Psychiatric update. Presented at the 139th annual meeting of the American Psychiatric Association, May, in Washington, D. C.

Gawin, F. H. (1986b) Neuroleptic reduction of cocaine-induced paranoia but not euphoria? *Psychopharmacol.* 90:142–143.

Gawin, F. H., Byck, R. & Kleber, H. D. (1985) Double-blind comparison of desipramine and placebo in chronic cocaine abusers. Presented at the 24th meeting of the American College of Neuropharmacology, December, in Kaanapali, Hawaii.

Gawin, F. H. & Kleber, H. D. (1984) Cocaine abuse treatment: Open pilot trial with desipramine and lithium carbonate. *Arch. Gen. Psychiat.* 41:903–910.

Gawin, F. H. & Kleber, H. D. (1985a) Neuroendocrine findings in chronic cocaine abusers. *Br. J. Psychiat.* 147:569–573.

Gawin, F. H. & Kleber, H. D. (1985b) Cocaine abuse in a treatment population: Patterns and diagnostic distractions. In: Kozel, N. J. & Adams, E. H. (Eds.), NIDA Res Mon Ser. *Cocaine use in America: Epidemiologic and clinical perspectives.* NIDA Research Monograph 61, DHHS pub. no. (ADM) 85-1414. Washington, D. C. : Government Printing Office, 182–192.

Gawin, F. H. & Kleber, H. D. (1986a) Abstinence symptomatology and psychiatric diagnosis in chronic cocaine abusers. *Arch. Gen. Psychiat.* 43: 107–113.

Gawin, F. H. & Kleber, H. D. (1986b) Pharmacological treatment of cocaine abuse. *Psych. Clin. N. Am.*

Gawin, F. H., Riordan, C. & Kleber, H. D. (1985) Methylphenidate use in non-ADD cocaine abusers—a negative study. *Am. J. Drug Alch. Abuse* 11:- 193–197.

Giannini, A. J., Malone, D. A., Giannini, M. C., Price, W. A. & Loiselle, R. H. (1986) Treatment of depression in chronic cocaine and phencyclidine abuse with desipramine. *J Clin Pharmacol.* 26: 211–214.

Goeders, N. E. & Smith, J. E. (1983) Cortical dopaminergic involvement in cocaine reinforcement. *Science* 221:773–775.

Gold, M. S., Pottash, A. L. C. & Annitto W. D. (1983) Cocaine withdrawal: Efficacy of tyrosine. Presented at the 13th annual meeting of the Society for Neuroscience, November, in Boston.

Gold, M. S., Washton, A. M. & Dackis, C. A. (1985) Cocaine abuse: Neurochemistry, phenomenology, and treatment. In: Kozel, N. J. & Adams, E. H. (Eds.), *Cocaine use in America: Epidemiologic and clinical perspectives.* NIDA Research Monograph 61, DHHS pub. no. (ADM) 85-1414. Washington, D. C.: Government Printing Office, 130–150.

Groppetti, A., Zambotti, F., Biazzi, A. & Mantegazza, P. (1974) Amphetamine and cocaine on amine turnover. In: Usdin, E. & Snyder, S. (Eds.), *Frontiers in catecholamine research.* New York: Pergamon Press, 917–925.

Johanson, C. E. (1984) Assessment of the dependence potential of cocaine in animals. In: Grabowski, J. (Ed.), *Cocaine: Pharmacology, effects, and treatment of abuse.* NIDA Research Monograph 50, DHHS pub. no. (ADM) 84-1326. Washington, D. C. : Government Printing Office, 54–71.

Jonsson, L. E., Gunne, L. M. & Anggard, E. (1969) Effects of alpha-methyltyrosine in amphetamine-dependent subjects. *Pharmacologia Clinica* 2:27–29.

Kalant, H. & Kalant, O. J. (1979) Death in amphetamine users: Causes and rates. In: Smith, D. E., Wesson, D. R., Buxton M. E., et al. (Eds.), *Amphetamine use, misuse, and abuse.* Boston: G. K. Hall.

Khantzian, E. J. (1983) Cocaine dependence, an extreme case and marked improvement with methylphenidate treatment. *Am. J. Psychiat.* 140:784–785.

Khantzian, E. J., Gawin, F. H., Riordan, C. & Kleber, H. D. (1984) Methylphenidate treatment of cocaine dependence—a preliminary report. *J. Subst. Abuse Treatment* 1:107–112.

Khantzian, E. J. & Khantzian, N. J. (1984) Cocaine addiction: Is there a psychological predisposition? *Psychiatric Annals* 14:753–759.

Kleber, H. D. & Gawin, F. H. (1984) Cocaine abuse: A review of current and experimental treatments. In: Grabowski, J. (ed.), *Cocaine: Pharmacology, effects, and treatment of abuse.* NIDA Research Monograph 50, DHHS pub. no. (ADM) 84-1326. Washington, D. C.: Government Printing Office, 111–129.

Kokkinidis, L. & Zacharko, R. (1980) Response sensitization and depression following long-term amphetamine treatment in a self-stimulation paradigm. *Psychopharmacology* 68:73–76.

Kramer, J. C., Fischman, V. S. & Littlefield, D. C. (1967) Amphetamine abuse patterns and effects of high doses taken intravenously. *JAMA* 201:305–309.

Lasagna, L., von Felsinger, J. M. & Beecher, H. K. (1955) Drug induced mood changes in man. I. Observations on healthy subjects, chronically ill patients, and postaddicts. *JAMA* 157:1020–1066.

Leith, N. J. & Barrett, R. J. (1976) Amphetamine and the reward system: Evidence for tolerance and post-drug depression. *Psychopharmacology* 46:19–25.

Lewin, L. (1924) *Phantastica.* Berlin: Verlag von Georg Stilke.

Maier, H. W. (1926) *Der Kokainismus.* Leipzig: George Thieme Verlag.

Nathanson, M. H. (1937) The central action of beta-aminopropylbenzene (Benzedrine). *JAMA* 108:528–531.

Post, R. M., Kopanda, R. T. & Black, K. E. (1976) Progressive effects of cocaine on behavior and central amine metabolism in rhesus monkeys: Relationship to kindling and psychosis. *Biol. Psychiat.* 11:403–419.

Resnick, R. B. & Resnick, E. B. (1984) Cocaine abuse and its treatment. *Psychiatr. Clin. North Am.* 7:713–728.

Ricuaurte, G. A., Schuster, C. R. & Seiden, L. S. (1980) Long-term effects of repeated methylamphetamine administration on dopamine and serotonin neurons in rat brain: A regional study. *Brain Res.* 193:153.

Rosecan, J. (1983) The treatment of cocaine abuse with imipramine, L-tyrosine, and L-tryptophan. Presented at the 7th World Congress of Psychiatry, July, in Vienna, Austria.

Rounsaville, R. J., Gawin, F. H. & Kleber, H. D. (1985) Interpersonal Psychotherapy (IPT) adapted for ambulatory cocaine abusers. *Am. J. Drug Alch. Abuse* 11:171–191.

Rowbotham, M., Jones, R. T., Benowitz, N. & Jacob, P. (1984) Trazodone-oral cocaine interactions. *Arch. Gen. Psychiat.* 41:895–899.

Schuster, C. R. & Fischman, M. W. (1985) Characteristics of human volunteering for a cocaine research project. In: Kozel, N. J. & Adams, E. H. (Eds.), *Cocaine use in America: Epidemiologic and clinical perspectives.* NIDA Research Monograph 61, DHHS pub. no. (ADM) 85-1414. Washington, D. C.: Government Printing Office, 158–170.

Seiden, L. (1984) Neurochemical toxic effects of psychomotor stimulants. Presented at the 23rd annual meeting of the American College of Neuropharmacology, December, in San Juan, Puerto Rico.

Siegel, R. K. (1982) Cocaine smoking. *J. Psychoact. Drugs* 14:321–337.

Siegel, R. K. (1985) New patterns of cocaine use: Changing doses and routes. In: Kozel, N. J. & Adams, E. H. (Eds.), *Cocaine use in America: Epidemiologic and clinical perspectives.* NIDA Research Monograph 61, DHHS pub. no. (ADM) 85-1414. Washington, D. C. Government Printing Office, 204–220.

Smith, D. E. (1969) The characteristics of dependence in high-dose methamphetamine abuse. *Int. J. Addict.* 4: 453–459.

Taylor, D. & Ho, B. T. (1977) Neurochemical effects of cocaine following acute and repeated injection. *J. Neurosci.* 3:95.

Taylor, D. L., Ho, B. T. & Fagan, J. D. (1979) Increased dopamine receptor binding in rat brain by repeated cocaine injection. *Commun. Psychopharmacol.* 3:137–142.

Tennant, F. (1985) Double-blind comparison of desipramine and placebo in withdrawal from cocaine dependence. In: Harris, L. S. (Ed.), *Problems of drug dependence.* NIDA Research Monograph, DHHS pub. no. (ADM) 76. Washington, D. C.: Government Printing Office.

Utena, H. (1966) Behavioral aberrations in methamphetamine intoxicated animals and chemical correlates in the brain. *Prog. Brain Res.* 21:1902.

Van Dyke, C., Ungerer, J., Jatlow, P. & Byck, R. (1982) Intranasal cocaine dose relationships of psychological effects and plasma levels. *Int. J. Psych. Med.* 12:1–13.

Watson, R., Hartmann, E. & Schildkraut, J. J. (1972) Amphetamine withdrawal: Affective state, sleep patterns and MHPG excretion. *Am. J. Psychiat.* 129:263–269.

Weiss, R. D., Mirin, S. M. & Michael, J. L. (1983) Psychopathology in chronic cocaine abusers. Presented at the 136th annual meeting of the American Psychiatric Association, May, in New York.

Woolverton, W. L., Kamien, J. B. & Kleves, M. S. (1987) Blockade of the discriminative stimulus effects of cocaine and of amphetamine in rhesus monkeys with the D_1 dopamine antagonist SCH 23390. *Pharmacologist* 29:158.

Wurmser, L. (1974) Psychoanalytic considerations of the etiology of compulsive drug use. *J. Am. Psychoanl. Assoc.* 22:820–843.

Yagi, B. (1963) Studies in general activity. II. The effect of methamphetamine. *Ann. Animal Psychol.* 13:37–47.

Yokel, R. A. & Wise, R. A. (1983) Increased lever pressing of amphetamine after pimozide in rats: Implications for a dopamine theory of reward. *Science* 221:773–774.

Index